Delivering the Government's Mental Health Policies

Services, staffing and costs

Jed Boardman and Michael Parsonage

ISBN13: 978 1 870480 72 7

Published by
The Sainsbury Centre for Mental Health
134–138 Borough High Street
London SE1 1LB
Tel: 020 7827 8300
Fax: 020 7827 8369
www.scmh.org.uk

The Sainsbury Centre for Mental Health (SCMH) is a charity that works to improve the quality of life for people with severe mental health problems. SCMH was founded in 1985 by the Gatsby Charitable Foundation, one of the Sainsbury Family Charitable Trusts, from which it receives core funding. SCMH is affiliated to the Institute of Psychiatry at King's College, London.

A charitable company limited by guarantee registered in England and Wales no. 4373019

Charity registration no. 1091156

Design: www.intertype.com

Printing: Ashford Overload

Contents

Executive Summary

Background

The National Service Framework for Mental Health (NSF-MH), published by the Department of Health in late 1999, set an ambitious ten-year agenda for improving mental health care in England. Subsequent policy statements and guidance, including NICE guidelines, have supplemented the Framework and added to the overall scale of the task.

This report assesses what needs to be done in delivering the key objectives of current mental health policy, organised around the seven standards of the NSF-MH, in terms of service provision, staffing and funding.

Because the NSF-MH and related documents are not always sufficiently explicit or prescriptive about how the stated standards should be achieved, much of the report consists of a detailed description of the individual services that are required for the delivery of policy. These specifications cover the full range of mental health provision, whether hospital-based or community-based, and include services provided in primary care as well as those of a specialist nature.

Building on these service specifications, the report then analyses what the delivery of policy implies at an aggregate level for the size of the mental health workforce and for the scale of public spending on mental health services.

In keeping with the coverage of the NSF-MH, the focus of the report is on the provision of mental health care for working-age adults (16–65 years) in England. Services for children and for older-age adults are therefore excluded. Also, in line with the planned ten-year timescale for implementation of the NSF-MH, the analysis relates to a set of services, with associated staffing and spending requirements, to be available in 2010/11.

The findings of this report have a variety of potential uses, locally as well as nationally. For example, the service specifications provide a detailed set of benchmarks which may be useful for the local planning of services and workforce needs.

Key findings

Services and staffing

Standard 1 – Mental health promotion and discrimination/exclusion

Little official guidance is available on the specification of services or staffing needs for standard 1 of the NSF-MH. Much may be accomplished by cross-cutting policies, but specific initiatives need to be housed in health and social services. Current good practice indicates that, at minimum, a mental health promotion team of eight staff is required for an average local population of 250,000 people.

Standards 2 & 3 – Primary care and access to services

For mental health services in primary care (standards 2 and 3), the report does not prescribe any particular model of service, as this is not defined in Government policy, but focuses instead on specific needs for medication and psychological therapies among people with common mental health problems. Improved access to psychological therapies will require approximately 11,000 psychological therapists at the primary care level, in addition to the 1,000 new graduate primary care mental health workers and 500 gateway workers announced in the NHS Plan of 2000.

Standards 4 & 5 – Services for people with severe mental illness – Community-based teams

The services required for people with severe mental illness (standards 4 and 5) are more clearly defined in official guidance. This particularly applies to the services provided by community-based teams (community mental health teams and the new specialist functional teams providing crisis resolution, assertive outreach and early intervention services). Our analysis suggests that nearly 18,000 additional community team care staff are needed by 2010/11 if the NSF-MH standards are to be implemented. This is an increase of around 80% on current numbers. The staffing gap is particularly large in the case of early intervention teams, where the numbers currently working are only about a fifth of the required level.

There is also a need to diversify the types of staff traditionally seen in community teams, including for example more pharmacists, dual diagnosis workers, employment specialists and support workers for people from BME communities.

A range of additional community services are required to augment the core community teams. Many of these may be supplied by the voluntary sector, including advice and information services, advocacy services, befriending and voluntary schemes, self-help and mutual aid groups and service user groups.

Standards 4 & 5 – Services for people with severe mental illness – Inpatient services

Community services must be backed up by good-quality acute inpatient services, supported by a range of residential accommodation and rehabilitation facilities. Projections for numbers of beds and residential places in 2010/11 were mainly taken from the National Beds Inquiry published by the Department of Health in 2000. The total number of care staff required for inpatient and residential units (excluding forensic units) in 2010/11 is estimated at around 85,000.

As with the community teams, there is a need to diversify the types of staff employed in these units, for example to improve medicines management and physical care for patients, to increase the therapies and activities available and to improve the social component of care.

Standards 4 & 5 – Services for people with severe mental illness – Day care and employment services

Day services are in need of reorganisation and should be closely allied to employment schemes. Service specifications and staff needs were based on recent official guidance on day services and the series of cross-departmental initiatives on social inclusion. About 3,500 staff are currently employed in day care and related services, which is only about a third of the required level.

Standards 4 & 5 – Services for people with severe mental illness – Forensic services

Forensic services were assessed separately. Because the capacity requirement for inpatient services is not well defined, current numbers of secure beds were used as the basis of the calculations, implying provision of 820 high secure beds and around 4,430 medium secure beds. Outside hospital, community forensic teams are in their infancy and need developing for the community management of offenders and those discharged from secure inpatient units.

Staffing needs for mental health services in prisons were examined and it is estimated that in a typical category B prison of 550 inmates an in-reach team of around 14 whole-time equivalent staff is required.

Standards 4 & 5 – Services for people with severe mental illness – Sub-speciality services

A series of sub-specialty mental health services are needed to provide services for working-age adults which are additional to the core community and inpatient services. These include general hospital liaison services, perinatal services, services for people with eating disorders and personality disorders and services for deaf people.

Standard 6 – Services for carers

Standard 6 of the NSF-MH covers services for carers. These are at presently poorly provided. For example, there are currently about 800 carer support workers in England, but more than double this number are needed by 2010/11.

Costs

Looking across mental health services as a whole, it is estimated that in order to implement the NSF-MH in full by 2010/11, aggregate staff numbers need to increase by 38% relative to the numbers employed in mental health care in 2005/06.

Allowing for non-pay inputs and for real increases in pay, the projected increase in staff numbers translates into a required increase in total public spending on mental health services between 2005/06 and 2010/11 of 53% in real terms (i.e. over and above general inflation). This is equivalent to an average real increase of 8.8% a year. (In comparison, an official estimate of the cost of the NSF-MH, published in the 2002 Wanless report on long-term health spending, implies that over the same period expenditure needs to rise at the even faster rate of 9.6% a year.)

An analysis of past spending shows that, between 1999/2000 (when the NSF-MH was published) and 2005/06, expenditure on mental health services increased in real terms by 47%, equivalent to an average rise of 6.7% a year. This was a substantial achievement and allowed considerable progress to be made in improving services along the path set by the NSF-MH.

On the other hand, even if expenditure continues to grow at this rate, it will be insufficient for the full implementation of policy by 2010/11. In addition, it seems unrealistic to assume that spending will in fact continue to rise so rapidly, particularly in the light of the Government's announced plans for a substantial slow-down in the growth of public spending as a whole after 2007/08.

A plausible assessment is that in 2010/11 funded capacity for adult mental health care is likely to be at around 80% of its required or target level. The implied shortfall of 20% should perhaps be seen as a measure of the very ambitious nature of the policy agenda that was set by the NSF-MH rather than as a sign of failure or under-achievement.

Conclusions

- Some of the present service models integral to the NSF-MH require more detailed specification, in particular those relating to mental health promotion and services in primary care. For secondary care the planning of services for the rehabilitation of those with severe mental illness and the interface with services for young people, those with learning difficulties (including autistic spectrum disorders) and those with alcohol and drug misuse require policy initiatives to promote their improvement.
- Importantly, the development of services and staff competencies should have as a central objective the promotion of social inclusion of people with mental health problems.
- There is a clear need to increase staff numbers in both professionally and non-professionally affiliated groups and attention should be paid to their recruitment, training and standards. The execution of roles and ways of working together should be examined as laid out in New Ways of Working, published by the Department of Health in 2005.
- The provision of evidence-based treatments, services and policy is crucial. An opportunity to monitor and evaluate the implementation of the NSF-MH standards may have been lost. There remains an urgent need to institute a robust evaluation of the effects of the modernisation of community services and assessment of the progress of NSF-MH standards. In addition, how much have we succeeded in delivering improved outcomes for mental health services and users?
- The NSF-MH set an ambitious agenda which is unlikely to be realised in full by 2010/11. This raises questions about priorities for the future and for the distribution of resources across England. If funds for mental health become more constrained and not all the objectives of policy can be delivered, how and where can any extra money be most sensibly used?
- There is a vision of services implicit in those aspects of policy that promote social inclusion, citizenship and rights, which are central to the lives of current and potential service users. A clear long-term strategy and sufficient resources, which are equitably distributed, should be made available to match this vision.
- The momentum gained and the present priority status for mental health services need to be maintained. This calls for a successor to the NSF-MH, setting out a clear plan for the future direction, standards, delivery and structure of mental health services, including a published analysis of the staffing and other resource implications.

Introduction

This report describes the findings of a major project undertaken by the Sainsbury Centre for Mental Health on the specification and costing of a mental health service which delivers the Government's key policy objectives for mental health. The report takes the seven standards of the *National Service Framework for Mental Health* (NSF-MH) (Department of Health, 1999) as the central component of this policy.

In November 2005 a discussion paper published by the Sainsbury Centre for Mental Health was sent out for consultation (Boardman & Parsonage, 2005). This contained an earlier version of the service descriptions outlined in the present report and comments were invited on how the specifications might be modified and refined, particularly with a view to achieving a broad consensus of professional and other opinions on a central model for a policy-compliant mental health service. A large number of responses were received, leading to a substantial strengthening of the analysis. We are very grateful to all those who commented during this consultation phase of the project.

The revised service specifications set out in this report are as far as possible based on published evidence, but as before it should be emphasised that they represent only one possible version of a mental health service that might deliver the objectives of current policy. It should also be noted that, on the whole, a conservative approach has been taken, avoiding the introduction of radical new models of service delivery or radical changes in staff roles. In this report we do not set out our vision for mental health services, rather we have taken the Government's policies and have attempted to put flesh on their bones by examining the services and workforce required to implement them and the associated costs of achieving this.

To our knowledge there has been only one officially published estimate of the cost of the NSF-MH, quoted in the Wanless Report (Wanless, 2002). This indicated that spending on mental health services would need to double in real terms between 2002/03 and 2010/11 to deliver the NSF-MH, but was otherwise low on detail. The present report has sought to expand on this by calculating on a service by service basis the workforce and cost implications of the NSF-MH and related policies.

Project parameters

The main questions addressed by the project were:

- What services are needed to implement the NSF-MH and related policies?
- How should these services be configured?
- What are the workforce implications?
- How much will it cost?

The project had two further central parameters:

- The focus of the analysis is on services for adults of working age (16-65 years) in England. This is in line with the coverage of the NSF-MH.
- The set of services described by the project is intended to be available by 2010/11. This is in line with the ten-year timescale set at the release of the NSF-MH in late 1999.

The project set itself two major challenges. The first was to base its specification of services on Government policy, including relevant NICE guidelines. The NSF-MH has been the central element of the Government's mental health policy for working-age adults and this project has used it as the main guide to outline the services and workforce required to deliver mental health care in England. There are however many other policy documents and official initiatives relating to mental health services for working-age adults and these have been used here to help specify the range of services required to deliver policy goals.

All services specified in this report are part of Government policy. Notwithstanding the details given in the NSF-MH and associated implementation guides and further policy statements, these documents are not always sufficiently explicit or prescriptive about the service structures and models that may be needed to deliver the seven NSF-MH standards. As a result, the specification of services described in this report has drawn not only on official guidance but also on local examples of good practice and on professional judgement.

The second challenge was, whenever possible, to base the figures for services and staffing on population needs supported by sound epidemiological data. Population-based figures have been used if available, but where these are not available figures based on the current use of services or official projections have been substituted.

Policy background

Mental health services in England have changed considerably over the past 20 years. Community services have developed, asylums have closed and mental health has become an NHS priority area for development (Boardman, 2005).

The present Government first set out its view of modern mental health services for adults of working age in the White Paper *Modernising Mental Health Services: Safe, sound and supportive* (Department of Health, 1998a). Importantly this announced the Government's intention to invest an additional £700 million in mental health services over three years and to create a National Service Framework for Mental Health (NSF-MH) for working-age adults. The White Paper built on already published documents detailing intended reforms to health and social services including: *Our Healthier Nation* (Department of Health, 1998b); *The New NHS: Modern and dependable* (Department of Health, 1997); *Modernising Social Services* (Department of Health, 1998c); and *A First Class Service: Quality in the new NHS* (Department of Health, 1998d).

The publication of the *National Service Framework for Mental Health* (Department of Health, 1999) set out for the first time a set of officially sanctioned minimum standards which mental health services were expected to attain. The *NHS Plan* (Department of Health, 2000a) amplified these by specifying the number of new community teams that were to be developed, linked developments with additional funding and reiterated that mental health was to be one of the three priority areas alongside cancer and coronary heart disease. The subsequent *Mental Health Policy Implementation Guide*

(Department of Health, 2001a) was published with the intention of supporting local implementation teams in the delivery of adult mental health policy and set out service specifications for crisis resolution/home treatment teams, assertive outreach teams and early intervention teams.

Subsequent developments suggested that increased funds for mental health were not always getting to the services that they were meant to support (The Sainsbury Centre for Mental Health, 2003) and other policy documents set out additional areas of development that were aligned to the NSF-MH, for example social inclusion (Social Exclusion Unit, 2004) and race equality (Department of Health, 2005a). The five-year review of the NSF-MH (Department of Health, 2004a) showed progress towards some of the targets but acknowledged that more needed to be done in some areas, that money had often been diverted to other services and that inequities of provision remained across the country.

The current plan for the development of adult mental health services in England is defined by the National Service Framework for Mental Health, NHS Plan and Policy Implementation Guides. To a large degree these have prescribed the development of services, particularly at the secondary care level, but it remains unclear precisely what an adult mental health service should look like, what staff and other resources are necessary to provide this and its costs.

The National Service Framework for Mental Health

The NSF-MH sets seven standards in five areas, to be delivered over a ten-year period:

Standard 1	Mental health promotion and discrimination/exclusion
Standards 2 & 3	Primary care and access to services.
Standards 4 & 5	Services for people with severe mental illness
Standard 6	Services for carers
Standard 7	Actions necessary to reduce suicides.

The NHS Plan

Chapter 14 (The Clinical Priorities) set out the details of services to be provided to support the NSF-MH. The priority was to ensure that people with severe and enduring mental health problems receive services that are more responsive to their needs. The Plan provided extra investment of over £300 million a year by 2003/04 to fast-forward the NSF-MH.

The NHS Plan also pointed out that by April 2001 there would be almost 500 extra secure beds, over 320 24-hour staffed beds, 170 assertive outreach teams and access to services 24 hours a day, seven days a week, for all those with complex mental health needs.

The priorities were set for primary care, early intervention in psychosis, crisis resolution, assertive outreach services, services for women, support for carers, high secure hospitals and prison services.

Policy Implementation Guides

The *Mental Health Policy Implementation Guide* (Department of Health, 2001a) was published with the intention of supporting local implementation teams in the delivery of adult mental health policy. Service specifications were set out for crisis resolution/home treatment teams, assertive outreach teams and early intervention teams and advice given on primary care mental health, mental health promotion, cultural sensitivity, gender sensitivity, involving and supporting service users and carers, and workforce needs assessment. Other specific Policy Implementation Guides (PIGs) have been published subsequently (Department of Health, 2002a; 2002b; 2002c; 2002d; Department of Health, 2003a; 2003b; 2003c; 2003d; Department of Health, 2004b; 2004c).

Other aspects of mental health policy

The social exclusion of people with mental health problems has featured in policy documents of several government departments including the Office of the Deputy Prime Minister Social Exclusion Unit's report on mental health and social exclusion (Social Exclusion Unit, 2004). The recommendations of the Social Exclusion Unit have been taken up by the National Institute for Mental Health in England (NIMHE) for implementation.

In addition, the Department for Work and Pensions (DWP) has been concerned with disability and benefit reform (HM Government, 2006) and the Department of Health has published guidelines on day services and vocational services (Department of Health/Department for Work and Pensions, 2006; Department of Health, 2006a). Specific groups have been given particular attention, including Black and ethnic minorities (Department of Health, 2003e; 2005a), prisoners (Department of Health/HM Prison Service, 2001), people with personality disorders (NIMHE, 2003), women (Department of Health, 2002e; 2006b) and carers (Department of Health, 2002f).

The Mental Health Act has been a controversial area for reform with the Government's original plans for a new Mental Health Act (Department of Health, 2004d) being abandoned in favour of amending the 1983 Act (Department of Health, 2006c).

The future workforce of the NHS has been a continuing concern (Department of Health, 1998e) and the problems of recruitment and retention in mental health services have been highlighted (Department of Health, 2001b; 2004e). A recent report outlined new ways of working for consultant psychiatrists and other professional groups in the mental health workforce (Department of Health, 2005b).

The NSF five-year review

The five-year review of the NSF-MH was published in 2004 (Department of Health, 2004a). In addition to reviewing the progress towards targets over the first five years, it set some priorities for the next five years:

- Inpatient care
- Dual diagnosis
- Social exclusion
- Ethnic minorities
- Care of long-term mental disorders
- Availability of psychological therapies
- Better information and information systems
- Workforce redesign with new roles for key staff.

It also put mental health services in the context of overall developments in health and social services: "We now need to plan for the next five years in a way that re-casts our NSF in line with the direction that the NHS as a whole is taking – towards patient choice, the care of long-term conditions and improved access to services" (Department of Health, 2004a).

Other broader policy initiatives

The policy initiatives for mental health should be set in the context of broader NHS policies, which were set out in the *NHS Plan* in 2000 (Department of Health, 2000a; Department of Health, 2004f). These included changes in funding arrangements and commissioning (Department of Health, 2003f; 2003g; 2004g; 2006d), increasing patient choice and patient and public involvement (Secretary of

State for Health, 2003, Department of Health, 2004h; 2005c). These have been associated with a focus of care outside hospitals (Secretary of State for Health, 2006) and the management of chronic disease (Department of Health, 2001c; 2005d; 2005e).

National Institute for Mental Health in England (NIMHE)

NIMHE was set up in 2002 to implement and develop Government mental health policy and its main sponsor is the Department of Health (Department of Health, 2001d). It is now part of the Care Services Improvement Partnership (CSIP), which supports improvement and development across a range of health and social services and local government. NIMHE has eight regional development centres through which the majority of their work is delivered and they host the Mental Health Research Network.

National Institute for Health and Clinical Excellence (NICE)

The National Institute for Clinical Excellence was established in England and Wales in 1999 to provide guidance to the NHS on health technologies (see Department of Health, 1997; Department of Health, 1998d). In April 2005 it combined with the Health Development Agency to form the National Institute for Health and Clinical Excellence (NICE) (see Department of Health, 2004h). NICE, an independent organisation, has now expanded its functions to provide national guidance on the promotion of good health and the prevention and treatment of ill health.

The Department of Health commissions NICE to develop guidance. Currently NICE produces three types of guidance:

- **Technology appraisals.** These are recommendations for the use of new and existing medicines and treatments. Existing appraisals of relevance to mental health conditions are computerised cognitive behavioural therapy, ECT, atypical antipsychotic drugs for schizophrenia and drugs used in mania.
- **Clinical guidelines.** These are recommendations for the appropriate treatment and care of people with specific diseases and conditions. Mental health conditions presently covered by these include: anxiety, depression, schizophrenia, eating disorders, post-traumatic stress disorders and deliberate self-harm.
- **Interventional procedures.** This guidance covers the safety and efficacy of interventional procedures used for diagnosis and treatment. There are currently none directly relevant to mental health services.

NICE is responsible for setting clear standards for treatments provided in the NHS. How health care organisations should respond to NICE guidance is set out in the Department of Health's *Standards for Better Health* (Department of Health, 2004i) and the standards which form the basis of the annual assessment of NHS organisations by the Healthcare Commission include requirements to conform to NICE guidance.

The project

The project described in this report has sought to define a mental health service that will deliver the policies, standards and guidelines outlined here and to quantify the staffing and expenditure needed to achieve this.

There were four main stages to the analysis. The first stage created a detailed specification of services, based on a consideration of what type and configuration of provision is implied by present policy and guidance. For some types of service, for example assertive outreach teams, this is explicit in the published guidance, while for others, for example in primary care, there are no explicit or agreed models. For these latter areas, we chose to focus on the resource requirements for provision of accepted treatments and services or on current examples of good practice. Use was made of NICE guidelines when specified standards of treatment were required for the analysis.

The second stage was to relate these service descriptions to needs for mental health care, as represented by the underlying epidemiological base. As far as possible, reference was made to population-based figures of existing rates of mental health conditions based on population surveys. In some cases this was not possible and usage figures or official projections were employed instead.

Third, the volumes of service provision generated by the first two stages of analysis were translated into matching workforce requirements disaggregated by type of staff (psychiatrists, psychologists, nurses, social workers etc.).

Finally, the projected staff numbers were converted into expenditure terms using appropriate pay rates and combined with estimated levels of spending on non-pay inputs so as to give a figure for total required expenditure in financial year 2010/11, covering all forms of mental health provision for adults of working age.

A schematic representation of these steps in the analysis is shown in Figure 1.

Figure 1: Steps in project analysis

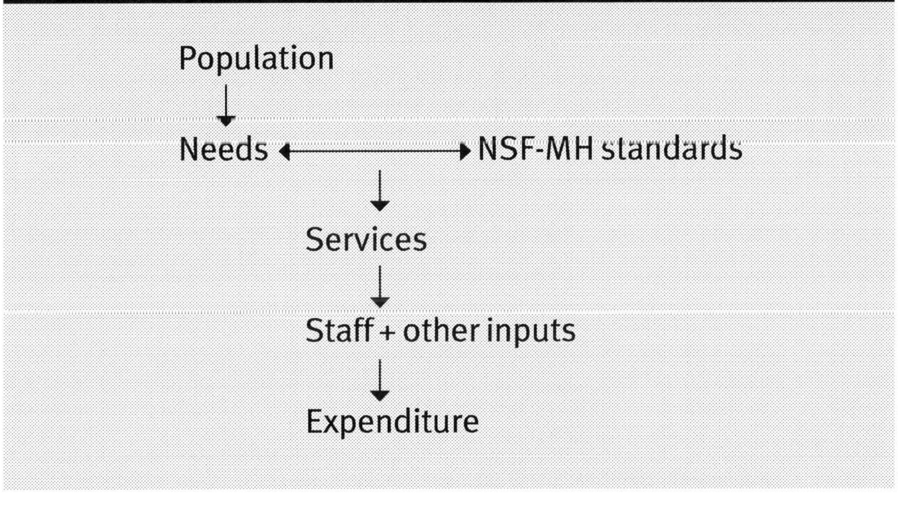

As Figure 1 shows, the end-product of the analysis is a quantified model of the mental health system. A feature of the model is that it can readily be re-calibrated to incorporate changed assumptions or data and so could be used, for example, to assess the workforce and expenditure implications of different levels or methods of service delivery. This is an important consideration given that the NSF-MH and its accompanying implementation guides are not always explicit about the models or structures of provision needed to deliver the seven standards. In addition, the model could be adapted using demographic and other data relating to a specific locality and thus serve as a local planning tool. We plan to explore possible options for taking forward the development of the analysis in these ways.

Population base

Population estimates for 2010 were used in the calculations for services and staffing as this is the year by which the NSF-MH standards are to be implemented. These estimates were based on the official census projections for 2010 (Government Actuary's Department, 2006). The projected total population for England in 2010 is 51,715,000, including 34,262,000 people (66.25%) aged 16–65 years. These figures represent the underlying population base used in our analysis.

For ease of presentation the detailed service specifications for each NSF-MH standard described in the report relate to a hypothetical catchment area with a total population of 250,000. It is assumed that this hypothetical locality is representative of England in all relevant respects, including demographic structure. From the figures given in the official census projections, the local population of 250,000 will therefore include 165,625 adults of working age in 2010 (Box 1).

Box 1: Census data for a catchment area of 250,000 people

	Year 2010
Total population	250,000
Aged 16–65 years	165,625
Men	82,822
Women	82,802

It is acknowledged that socio-demographic characteristics and other determinants of the need for mental health care vary greatly across the country and so the findings of this study will need adjustment if they are to be used in a local context. This may be particularly relevant in rural areas where the assessment of need may be difficult, not least because of the considerable changes that these communities have undergone in recent years, the tendency to find hidden deprivation alongside apparent areas of affluence and the difficulty in readily identifying vulnerable groups (Mind, 2004). In addition, the development of services in these areas may be hampered by problems of workforce development owing to historically poor recruitment and retention of a skilled workforce, the existing infrastructure and the need to develop service models that address geography, distance, communications and a dispersed population. It is recommended that particular attention is paid to assessing need and the development of services in rural areas (Mind, 2004).

1 Standard 1 Mental health promotion and discrimination/exclusion

Standard 1

Health and social services should:

- promote mental health for all, working with individuals and communities
- combat discrimination against individuals and groups with mental health problems, and promote their social inclusion.

(Department of Health, 1999)

What type of service?

There are no nationally accepted models for mental health promotion or guidance for these services within health and social services. Some guidance is now available for improving the physical care of people with severe mental illness (Department of Health, 2006e). Much of the expenditure on promotion is likely to fall to non-health agencies, such as departments concerned with education or employment, and the costs falling on these departments are outside the scope of this project. Our estimates focus on the costs of services provided by the NHS and local authority social services departments (or voluntary agencies contracted to these).

In 2004, **mentality** undertook a national survey into the state of public mental health practice and found examples of good practice in mental health in local areas (**mentality**, 2005). The survey noted that individuals working in this field identified a lack of funding and a lack of local commitment to public mental health work.

Epidemiological and evidence base

At present there are no epidemiological figures that are of assistance in calculating the requirements for mental health promotion. In addition, direct evidence for the effectiveness of mental health promotion strategies is lacking, although there is indirect evidence concerned with the processes and interventions likely to produce behaviour and attitude change (Wardle & Steptoe, 2005; Abraham & Michie, 2005).

In view of these lacunae we have used a survey of existing provision to assist us to calculate the staffing figures for health service provision of mental health promotion initiatives. In addition to the survey detailed above, **mentality** asked 16 mental health promotion leads in England about current spending in this area. The survey revealed that those primary care trusts (PCTs) most active in this area had:

- 1.5 WTE mental health promotion and co-ordinator posts
- 1.5 WTE workers to promote mental health within families
- 1.5 WTE development workers to co-ordinate self-help groups for people with mental health problems.

In addition, there was a range of programmes and associated budgets. These included: training, locality networks for professionals with a mental health promotion role, mental health promotion and employment, physical activity, and mental health promotion for specific at-risk groups.

Staffing and service configuration

In 2005 there were 302 PCTs in England, covering an average population of 164,000 people. The staffing numbers noted in the **mentality** survey have been adjusted for a 250,000 population and are shown in Box 2. Additional sessional time has been added from a public health specialist in the field of health promotion. We have also followed the suggestions of the British Psychological Society Report (2004) which assumes that clinical psychologists have a strong role to play through the application of community psychology knowledge and approaches and that health psychologists have an important role in developing strategies likely to impact on health beliefs and evaluating the impact of these strategies.

Box 2: Health promotion staffing for a total population of 250,000

Staff	WTE
Mental health promotion specialists	2.3
Mental health family specialists	2.3
Self help/voluntary services co-ordinators	2.3
Public health specialist	0.2
Health psychologist	0.5
Clinical psychologist	0.5
Total	**8.1**

2 Standards 2 & 3
Primary care and access to services

Standard 2

Any service user who contacts their primary health care team with a common mental health problem should:

- have their mental health needs identified and assessed
- be offered effective treatments, including referral to specialist services for further assessment, treatment and care if they require it.

Standard 3

Any individual with a common mental health problem should:

- be able to make contact round the clock with the local services necessary to meet their needs and receive adequate care
- be able to use NHS Direct, as it develops, for first-level advice and referral on to specialist helplines or to local services.

(Department of Health, 1999)

What type of service?

Knowledge accrued over the years indicates that general practitioners (GPs) see and deal with the bulk of people with common mental disorders (predominantly syndromes of anxiety and depression) and a relatively small proportion (10–15%) are passed to secondary care. The GP and practice nurse have been seen as the mainstay of the delivery of mental health treatments with variable input from mental health specialists, in particular counsellors.

Recent changes to the GP contract and the introduction of the Quality and Outcome Framework (QOF) have given some emphasis to the physical care of people with mental illness, case finding for people with depression who have diabetes or ischaemic heart disease and the structured assessment of the severity of depressive disorders. This places potential improvements in mental health care in primary care within the delivery of general medical services. However, beyond this there is no clear model or consensus for the organisation and delivery of mental health services at the primary care level. It is however clear that the current management of depression in primary care is not satisfactory (Simon & von Korff, 1995; Scott, 2006). A systematic review of organisational interventions in primary care (Gilbody *et al.*, 2003) suggests some benefit from the use of 'collaborative care', which, whilst in practice varying in content, may be broadly characterised by being multifaceted and using new staff and new ways of working. Much of the evidence from these approaches comes from the USA and little from the UK.

In the absence of a clear model for delivering mental health interventions, we decided to adopt an approach which identified the main types of intervention for common mental disorders and to cost these. The two major forms of treatment delivered in primary care are medication and psychological therapies. There is a good evidence base for drug treatments in depression and anxiety and for a range of psychological therapies, in particular cognitive behavioural therapy (CBT) (NICE, 2004a; 2004b; Roth & Fonagy, 2004). Access to psychological therapies is highlighted as a priority area in the NSF five-year review and pilots for evaluating the delivery of CBT have begun in two sites in England.

In our calculations we have chosen to use CBT as the central intervention for common mental disorders, but acknowledge that other psychological approaches will be required and that a range of individual, group and systemic approaches will be desirable in a psychological therapy service for any one district. We also acknowledge that a comprehensive psychological therapy service will cover primary and secondary care and will have a range of providers.

Epidemiological base

Two main sources of prevalence figures are of relevance:

1. **General population surveys**
   The Office for National Statistics (ONS) (previously Office of Population Censuses and Surveys – OPCS) surveys of psychiatric morbidity in Great Britain (Meltzer *et al.*, 1995; Singleton *et al.*, 2001) indicate that the prevalence of common mental health problems (referred to as 'neurotic disorders' in the OPCS report) in adults aged 16–65 years in England is about 160 per 1,000 population. Thus 26,500 adults have common mental health problems in a population of 165,625.

   The rate of onset for common mental health problems was 6% in the 2000–2001 follow-up study (Singleton & Lewis, 2003). This means that there are likely to be 9,940 adults who develop new common mental health problems in a total population of 250,000 in one year.

2. **From surveys of people consulting in general practice**
   The most recent estimates are shown in Box 3, taken from Boardman *et al.* (2004). As the rates for the disorders are based on those consulting in general practice the denominator has been adjusted to reflect that approximately 65% of the people on a GP's list will consult in one year, i.e. 107,656 people in an adult population of 165,625.

Box 3: Number of adults aged 16–65 years in a total population of 250,000 consulting with depression and anxiety in primary care

DSM-IV disorder	Rate per 1,000 consulters	Number consulting
Major depression	107	11,519
Minor depression	44	4,737
Total depression	–	16,256
Anxiety disorder[1] (single diagnosis)	52	5,598

[1]Includes generalised anxiety disorder (GAD), panic disorder, agoraphobia and social phobia

The overall figures are very similar to those of the general population, but it is known that many people with mental health problems do not consult their GPs. The primary care figures give the rates for people with new and chronic disorders seen in general practice and can be placed against the actual needs for treatment measured in the same individuals as surveyed. These figures have thus been used to calculate the numbers of people requiring medication and psychological therapy in general practice over a 12-month period.

Calculations for depression

In the Boardman *et al.* (2004) study 65% of the people with depression had developed this during the previous year (they had new onsets of depression during that year, with many having experienced previous episodes). The study judged CBT to be suitable for 55% of the consulters with depression and antidepressant medication to be suitable for 70%.

Thus for a catchment area of 165,625 adults (107,656 consulting adults) there are 10,566 new onsets of depression per year (65% of 16,256). The number of people who require antidepressant medication and/or CBT in a catchment area of 165,625 will vary depending on the assumptions made.

If 70% of people with new onsets of depression who see their GP require antidepressant medication then 7,396 people will require these drugs. But not all people who have depression and are seen by the GP have this detected: on average about 60% of this is detected. Thus if only those who are detected and who need medication are given it, then the figure reduces to 4,438 (see Box 4).

The estimates for CBT are more difficult to make as it is uncertain how many people will require CBT in addition to, or instead of, medication. To calculate the numbers who need CBT and the number of therapists required, several assumptions have been made:

1. CBT will be given to those who do not adequately recover after being given antidepressants. This is in line with NICE depression guidelines. Approximately 60% of people recover after antidepressants: thus 40% will require CBT.
2. People will require 12 sessions of CBT over a 12-week period. This is based on an average of the figures given in the NICE depression guidelines, which recommend 6–8 sessions for mild depression and 16–20 sessions for moderate or severe depression.
3. If a therapist sees four clients per day for CBT, then a therapist may have a client list size of 20 people at any one time. Assuming that, on average, the sessions last for 12 weeks, then there will be four 12-week blocks available per year in which to conduct therapy. Thus a maximum of 80 people (4x20) can be seen by each therapist during a year.

These estimates are summarised in Box 4.

Box 4: Estimates for provision of antidepressant medication and CBT in primary care for depression

	Medication	CBT
Number of people with new onsets of depression seen in general practice over one year	10,566	10,566
Need (based on Boardman *et al.*, 2004)	70%	55%
Total number of people with new onsets in population of 165,625 who have need	7,396	5,811
Total number who have need if assume only 60% detected	4,438	3,487
Total number needing CBT if 40% do not recover with antidepressants only	–	2,324
Number needing CBT if only 60% detected and 40% do not recover with antidepressants	–	1,395

Thus for CBT:

❖ If all those people with new onsets of depression who do not recover after antidepressants are given CBT, then *29 therapists will be required* (2,324 divided by 80).

❖ If all those people with new onsets of depression who are detected and who do not recover after antidepressants are given CBT, then *17.4 therapists will be required* (1,395 divided by 80).

Calculations for anxiety

In the Boardman *et al.* (2004) study 47% of the people with anxiety had developed this during the previous year. The study judged CBT to be suitable for 79% of the consulters with anxiety and antidepressant medication (SSRIs) to be suitable for 60%.

Thus for a catchment area of 165,625 adults there are 2,631 new cases of anxiety per year (47% of 5,598). 1,597 of these people (or 947 if we consider only those who are detected) who have new onsets of anxiety will require antidepressant medication (Box 5).

Box 5: Estimates for provision of antidepressant medication and CBT in primary care for anxiety

	Medication	CBT
Number of people with new onsets of anxiety seen in general practice over one year	2,631	2,631
Need (based on Boardman *et al.*, 2004)	60%	79%
Total number of people with new onsets in population of 165,625 who have need	1,579	2,078
Total number who have need if assume only 60% detected	947	1,247

For CBT the assumptions made are:

1. CBT may be given at the same time as medication for people with anxiety. There are no clear guidelines about the timing of a combination of the two types of therapy.
2. People will require 12 sessions of CBT over a 12-week period. NICE guidelines recommend 7–14 hours of CBT for panic disorder and 16–20 hours for generalised anxiety disorder.
3. If any therapist sees four clients per day for CBT, then a therapist may have a client list size of 20 people at any one time. If the sessions last for 12 weeks, thus giving four 12-week blocks per year, a maximum of 80 people in total can be seen by each therapist per year.

These estimates are summarised in Box 5.

Thus for CBT:

1. If all those people with new onsets of anxiety are given CBT then *26 therapists will be required* (2,078 divided by 80).
2. If all those people with new onsets of anxiety who are detected are given CBT then *15.6 therapists will be required* (1,247 divided by 80).

The figures for new cases of depression can be combined with those for new cases of anxiety to give the total amount of medication and CB therapists required (Box 6).

Box 6: Total need for medication and cognitive behavioural therapists in primary care

	Total new cases	**Number in population of 165,625 who need treatment**		**Number of CB therapists**	
		Maximum If treat all people with new onsets who are in need	**Minimum** If treat people with new onsets in need, who are detected	**Maximum** If treat all people with new onsets who are in need	**Minimum** If treat people with new onsets in need, who are detected
Medication					
Anxiety	2,631	1,579	947	–	–
Depression	10,566	7,396	4,438	–	–
Total	**13,197**	**8,975**	**5,385**	–	–
CBT					
Anxiety	2,631	2,078	947	26	15.6
Depression	10,566	2,324	1,395	29	17.4
Total	**13,197**	**4,402**	**2,342**	**55**	**33**

Grossed up to the national level, these figures indicate that around 2.7 million people will consult their GP with new cases of depression or anxiety each year and a third of these should receive CBT. Current figures indicate that, among people consulting their GP with mental health problems, only about 1% receive CBT, 3% receive some other form of psychotherapy and a further 4% receive counselling (Layard *et al.*, 2006). A very substantial increase in the availability of talking therapy is therefore required. In contrast, the estimates for required levels of medication are broadly in line with current levels of provision.

There are some limitations to these estimates:

❖ ***The calculations only include people with new onsets of depression and anxiety.***

Depression may be best considered as a chronic disorder (Scott, 2006; von Korff & Goldberg, 2001). Many of the new onsets included in these figures had experienced previous episodes, but those omitted had long-term conditions and thus will require intervention over longer periods. Whilst this long-term group was not considered here they may be absorbed to some degree by the therapists suggested here.

The number of clients seen per day was estimated as four, but it may be possible to increase this to five to allow additional clients to be seen for 'booster' sessions because of their fluctuating chronic disorders or their relapsing conditions. However this does highlight the need to consider the system to deliver these therapies and the use of additional staff to assist in the management of chronic conditions. Some of these staff may be existing primary care workers who already provide input into the care of people with depression and anxiety, but additional workers may be required such as the primary care mental health workers (Department of Health, 2003c).

❖ ***They only focus on those people with depression and anxiety.***

These groups overlap as they contain people with mixed anxiety and depression. In the Boardman *et al.*, (2004) figures used in the calculations 45% of those with depression also had an anxiety disorder. The figures for anxiety disorders used in the calculations were for people who only had an anxiety disorder, thus avoiding double counting. Other related conditions, such as obsessive compulsive disorders, post-traumatic stress disorder (PTSD) and eating disorders have not been separately included in the calculations, despite being studied in Boardman *et al.* (2004). However, over 70% of the people identified in the study with these disorders also had a depressive disorder and are thus included in the above calculations. These groups will require mainly psychological interventions. However, they may present complex problems, emphasising the need to have well-trained and competent therapists with sufficient experience as well as adequate supervision.

❖ ***Other psychological therapies (e.g. counselling, psychodynamic psychotherapy, family and couple therapy) are not included.***

These will be required for some people with specific needs and form part of a comprehensive psychological therapies service. Not all people respond to CBT and other approaches will be required.

❖ ***Other means of delivering psychological therapy are not considered.***

These may include computerised methods and group approaches. The NICE guidelines suggest the use of approaches such as bibliotherapy, self-help and computerised CBT which may be ways of reducing the number who require one-to-one CBT, but there are no algorithms to help calculate these numbers. The CB therapists would have a role in assessing patients and introducing them to these approaches.

If CBT is to be provided for all those who need it in general practice, the staffing figures may be made up of the types of mental health worker outlined in Box 7.

Box 7: Proposed therapists required for primary care

Type of therapist	For 55 CB therapists
Clinical psychologist	27
CB therapist	22
CBT nurse therapist	6

The higher figure for psychological therapists has been used as it is assumed that the services would wish to treat all those people in need who present to the GP. The CB therapist is presumed to be specifically trained and paid at the same rate as counsellors who already work in primary care.

If 55 therapists are required for a total population of 250,000, 11,377 are required for the whole of England. In addition to these, the 1,000 new primary care mental health workers planned for primary care will still be required (Department of Health, 2003c). Five hundred gateway workers are also required for England (2.5 per 250,000 population) (Department of Health, 2003d).

How does this compare to other estimates?

In a recent paper delivered to a Cabinet Office seminar, Layard (2005, 2006) estimated that 10,000 cognitive behavioural therapists are required to provide adequate services for anxiety and depression.

Summary

In this chapter we elected to focus on the medication and psychological therapies required to meet the needs of those with anxiety and depression who present to primary care personnel. The associated staffing needs are considerable. No assumptions have been made about the specific means of delivering the psychological therapies. Further thought needs to be given to the types of mental health personnel required, their training and the most effective means and systems of delivering these therapies and their quality assurance.

3 Standards 4 & 5 Services for people with severe mental illness

Standard 4

All mental health service users on CPA should:

- ❖ receive care which optimises engagement, anticipates or prevents a crisis, and reduces risk
- ❖ have a copy of a written care plan which:
  - – includes the action to be taken in a crisis by the service user, their carer, and their care co-ordinator
  - – advises their GP how they should respond if the service user needs additional help
  - – is regularly reviewed by their care co-ordinator
- ❖ be able to access services 24 hours a day, 365 days a year.

Standard 5

Each service user who is assessed as requiring a period of care away from their home should have:

- ❖ timely access to an appropriate hospital bed or alternative bed or place, which is:
  - – in the least restrictive environment consistent with the need to protect them and the public
  - – as close to home as possible
- ❖ a copy of a written after care plan agreed on discharge which sets out the care and rehabilitation to be provided, identifies the care co-ordinator, and specifies the action to be taken in a crisis.

(Department of Health, 1999)

What type of service?

In comparison to services in primary care, specialist mental health services are more clearly prescribed in the NHS Plan and Implementation Guides. The following chapters on Standards 4 and 5 cover community-based teams (Chapter 4), inpatient services (including aftercare accommodation) (Chapter 5) and day care services (Chapter 6). However, it is recognised that these secondary care services must be complemented by forensic services (Chapter 7) and other sub-speciality services, for example perinatal and eating disorder services (Chapter 8).

Epidemiological base

The population figures for these standards may be based on the OPCS and ONS surveys (Meltzer *et al.*, 1995, Singleton *et al.*, 2001), Boardman *et al.* (2004) and estimates of mental illness from *Keys to Engagement* (The Sainsbury Centre for Mental Health, 1998) (see Box 8).

Box 8: Estimates of mental health problems in the population

	Prevalence rate	Number of working-age adults in a total population of 250,000
From OPCS/ONS		
Neurosis	160 per 1,000 adult population	26,500
Psychosis	4 per 1,000 adult population	662.5
Alcohol dependence	47 per 1,000 adult population	7,784
Drug dependence	22 per 1,000 adult population	3,644
From Boardman *et al.* (2004)		
Total non-psychotic mental illness in general practice	278 per 1,000 adult population (consulting)	29,928
From *Keys to Engagement* (SCMH, 1998)		
Severe mental illness	20–40 per 1,000 general population	7,500 (5,000–10,000)
Severe and enduring mental illness	3–15 per 1,000 adult population	1,491 (497–2,484)
Severe and enduring mental illness, difficult to engage	0.14–2.0 per 1,000 adult population	177 (23–331)

4 Standards 4 & 5 Community-based teams

Community mental health teams (CMHTs)

The Mental Health Policy Implementation Guide for CMHTs (Department of Health, 2002a) views these teams as the mainstay of the system and the core around which newer services are developed. They should offer people short-term contact services and continuing treatment, care and monitoring. Their functions include:

- work with primary care to provide a single point of entry
- assessment
- a multidisciplinary team approach
- regular review, including multidisciplinary and multi-agency review
- a range of interventions
- liaison with other parts of the health system and other agencies
- provision of discharge and transfer arrangements.

The Mental Health Policy Implementation Guide (PIG) for CMHTs recommends that each CMHT serve a population of 10,000 – 60,000 depending on the local levels of morbidity and travelling distances. It suggests a staffing of eight whole-time equivalent (WTE) care co-ordinators, each with a maximum caseload of 35 people, and a maximum caseload for the team as a whole of 300–350. The suggested staff mix is:

3–4 community psychiatric nurses (CPNs) }
2–3 approved social workers (ASWs) } Care co–ordinators
1–1.5 occupational therapists (OTs) }
1–1.5 clinical psychologists
1 consultant psychiatrists
1–1.5 other medical staff
1–3 support workers
1–1.5 secretaries
Reception staff
IT and audit support

For the purposes of the present calculations it is assumed that:

1. CMHTs need to cover two separate functions: assessment and continuing care.
2. Most assessments will be requested by primary care.
3. Users needing continuing care will be those with severe and enduring mental illness.
4. The caseload per team is 325. This is based on a *maximum* caseload size as opposed to an *ideal* size.

When considering caseload management and supervision a profile of the clinician's individual caseload may be assessed using one of the caseload profiling tools such as that developed by the NIMHE South West Development Centre (NIMHE, 2005a). This tool allows the practitioner to rate his/her caseload using three domains: case type, level of input into the case and the client's risk profile.

For the continuing care element of the team

If there are 1,491 people with severe and enduring mental illness in an adult population of 165,625 and each CMHT has a caseload of 325, then 4.5 CMHTs are required for a total population of 250,000. Thus, for this local population, if care co-ordinators are to have a caseload of no more than 35, then 42.6 staff (1,491 divided by 35) are required to look after this group of users, all of whom are assumed to be on CPA. The PIG assumes that only 280 of the 350 will be on enhanced CPA, but this may be optimistic as in this case all the users have severe and enduring mental illness, thus all ought to be on enhanced CPA. If care co-ordinators are to take on additional service users who are not on CPA then additional staff will be required.

For the assessment element of the team

A possible 29,928 users of CMHT services are seen in primary care. About 55% of these are new cases each year (based on Boardman *et al.*, 2004) and the referral rate from primary care is around 20%. This means that 3,591 people with new onsets will be referred each year.

Thus 798 people will be referred to each of the 4.5 teams each year (which equates to 16 per week or 3–4 per day). If we assume that one assessment can be done by a member of staff each day and additional follow-up consultations will be required, then four extra staff are needed for this component of the team. But extra staff will also be required to cover annual and study leave and an additional 28.4% staff are needed to cover this (see Chapter 5 [inpatient services] for a justification of these calculations). Thus, a total of five additional staff is required for the assessment component of the team.

Taking these two basic estimates and considering the staffing recommendations made by the PIG, the staffing for each team and for the population of 250,000 may look like that outlined in Box 9.

Box 9: WTE staff required for a total population of 250,000 – CMHTs

Staff	WTE per CMHT	Total staff for 250,000 total population (i.e. for 4.5 teams)
For continuing care	Total = 9.5	Total = 42.75
CPNs	5.0	22.5
Social workers	2.8	12.6
OTs	1.7	7.65
For assessment	Total = 5	Total = 22.5
CPNs	3	13.5
Social workers	2	9.0
Other professional staff	Total = 8.5	Total = 38.25
Consultants	1	4.5
Other medical staff	2	9.0
Clinical psychologists	1	4.5
Team leaders	1	4.5
Pharmacists	0.5	2.25
Dual diagnosis workers	1	4.5
Learning difficulties workers	1	4.5
Employment leads	1	4.5
Non-professionally affiliated staff	Total = 7.44	Total = 33.5
Pharmacy technicians	0.44	2.0
Psychology assistants	1	4.5
Support workers	See section on support workers	
Employment specialist workers	1	4.5
BME support workers	1	4.5
Administration staff	4	18.0
Total staff	**30.44**	**137.0**

There are several groups of workers included in the team that are additional to the usual complement of staff:

1. **Pharmacists**. Whilst there was little mention of pharmacists in the NSF-MH, subsequent policy documents have indicated their important role in improving medicines management (Department of Health 2000b; 2004j; Audit Commission, 2002). Within this role they should form partnerships with users and carers, work alongside other professionals in the team, support extended prescribing and contribute to the re-design of the workforce (Department of Health, 2005b; 2005f) The need for training of clinicians in medicines management was identified in the David Bennett inquiry (Department of Health, 2005a). Pharmacists, supported by pharmacy technicians, have a role to play in each of the community teams, for example, in reviewing medication (CPA and clinics), medicines information, supporting and informing patients and their carers, staff support, advice and education, supply of medicines, and liaison with GPs and community pharmacists about shared care prescribing. 0.5 WTE pharmacists have been added per team, with support from two pharmacy technicians across the teams.

2. **Dual diagnosis workers**. These would be professionally affiliated staff with the requisite training and experience in working with people with substance misuse and severe mental illness (Department of Health, 2002c). One such worker is required per team.

3. **Learning difficulties workers**. It is recognised that some people in contact with CMHTs will have learning difficulties or autism spectrum disorders. One member of staff has been added who will provide assessment for this group, support to other team members and liaison with local learning difficulty services.

4. **Employment leads**. The addition of this professional is recommended in recent guidance on vocational services for people with severe mental health problems (Department of Health/ Department for Work and Pensions, 2006) (see section on vocational services in Chapter 6). The role could be carried out by any mental health professional with the appropriate skills and experience, but may be suitable for those with an occupational therapy background.

In addition to the professionally affiliated staff, there are other groups of additional staff required in CMHTs:

5. **Psychology assistants**. These are additional staff to support the work of the clinical psychologist (British Psychological Society, 2004).

6. **Support workers**. A detailed discussion of the role of support workers, their numbers and distribution across the teams is set out later in this chapter. The numbers proposed for each team are based on the figures given in the Workforce Action Team (WAT) report for Support, Time and Recovery (STR) workers (Department of Health, 2001b). The role of these workers is set out in the relevant PIG (Department of Health, 2003a).

7. **Support workers for those from BME communities**. The role of this group of workers is set out in the relevant PIG (Department of Health, 2004b). The precise number of these workers for each team is difficult to estimate as this will depend on the size of the local BME community. One worker per team is assumed at this stage.

8. **Employment specialist workers**. The addition of this group of workers is recommended in the recent guidance on vocational services for people with severe mental health problems (Department of Health/Department for Work and Pensions, 2006).

9. **Administrative staff.** The number of administrative staff includes three secretaries and one receptionist per team.

In total, 931 teams are required for England with 28,340 total staff (24,519 care staff) and a caseload of 302,533 people with severe and enduring mental illness (out of an estimated range of 102,809 – 513,840). If greater coverage is required then the staffing estimates will inevitably increase.

How does this compare to other estimates?

The Durham Adult Mental Health (AMH) Service mapping data (Centre for Public Mental Health, Durham University, 2006) is the most comprehensive database of mental health services in England presently available and will be used, where relevant, to compare with our estimates. In Spring 2006 the Durham AMH mapping data reported 826 teams (one per 38,868 adult population) with 13,502 care staff (Centre for Public Mental Health, Durham University, 2006). In 2003 the CMHTs had a total caseload of 309,893 (mean of 373 per team) (Glover *et al.*, 2004).

Assertive outreach teams (AOTs)

Assertive outreach teams aim to support people with severe and enduring mental health problems who do not otherwise maintain contact with services. They were established to keep people out of hospital by giving them intensive support in the community for as long as is needed.

The Mental Health Policy Implementation Guide (MHPIG) (Department of Health, 2001a) suggests that each team covers a total population of 250,000 and that each team should have 90 service users at any one time with an ideal 10:1 ratio of users to care co-ordinators. The team should be made up of CPNs, ASWs, OTs, a clinical psychologist, a consultant psychiatrist and other medical staff.

If we assume that there are 177 people with severe and enduring mental illness who are difficult to engage (see Box 8), and thus suitable for assertive outreach, in a total population of 250,000 and that there will be a 10:1 users to staff ratio, then 17.7 care co-ordinator staff will be needed.

As with the CMHTs some additional workers have been placed in the teams. These are the same as for the CMHTs but no additional professional has been added as the employment lead. This role may be carried out by one of the existing members of the team.

The appropriate staffing for the team is shown in Box 10.

Box 10: WTE staff required for a total population of 250,000 – Assertive outreach teams (AOTs)	
Consultant psychiatrists	0.5
Other medical staff	1
Clinical psychologists	1
Team managers	1 } Total
CPNs	11.5 } care
OTs	2 } co-ordinators
Social workers	3.2 } = 17.7
Support workers	See section on support workers (p35)
Pharmacists	0.5
Pharmacy technicians	0.3
Psychology assistants	0.5
BME support workers	1
Employment specialists	1
Dual diagnosis workers	1
Admin. staff	1.5
Total	**26.0**

This means that by 2010 for the total England population there should be 207 teams with a total staff of 5,382 (4,906 care staff) and total caseload of 36,639 people.

How does this compare to other estimates?

The NHS Plan set a target of 220 assertive outreach teams. In Spring 2006 the Durham mapping data reported 251 teams (one per 127,910 adult population) with 2,551 care staff (8.5 per 100,000 adult population) plus 35 in CMHTs (Centre for Public Mental Health, Durham University, 2006). This suggests that there are sufficient numbers of teams, but inadequate numbers of staff.

Crisis resolution teams (CRTs)

Crisis resolution and home treatment teams (CRTs) were established to offer immediate support to people with severe mental health problems in a crisis. They aim to provide an alternative to inpatient admission and to 'gatekeep' admissions to hospital. They give short-term, intensive treatment and support during the crisis period to those who are not admitted to hospital.

The MHPIG (Department of Health, 2001a) does not specify how many CRTs are needed per unit of population. It suggests each team should have a caseload of 20 to 30 service users at any one time.

The staffing levels suggested are: 14 designated named workers per team (team leader plus up to 13 others) which include CPNs, ASWs, OTs, psychologists, support workers, medical staff (consultant and staff grade) and an administrative assistant.

To calculate the staffing for one of these teams we need to know:

1. **The likely number of crises occurring over a unit of time.** One of the purposes of a CRT is to provide an alternative to admission, thus the overall numbers of admissions should provide a guide to the number of possible crises (as the team should assess all these if they are to provide the 'gateway' to acute inpatient units). In 2001/2002 there were 120,994 admissions to psychiatric hospitals in England (HES data from www.dh.gov.uk). This equates to 608 per 250,000 total population per year. Thus there are likely to be 608 crises in the 250,000 catchment area (or 12 per week, 1.7 per day). If the team operates over 24 hours and this is split into three eight-hour periods then six people will be needed to assure that two workers are available to do assessments at any time.
2. **Length of time in contact with CRT.** This is more difficult to calculate, but if a month period is considered, then in week one 12 people will be seen, half of whom are still seen after one week when a further 12 arrive (total 18 people). In week 3 these are halved again and a further 12 added (3 + 6 + 12 = 21 people) and the same happens in week 4 (1 + 3 + 6 + 12 = 22 people). This would be in the range of service users suggested by the PIG (20 – 30). Thus the PIG estimates may be used and a maximum 30 patient team caseload assumed. It will also be assumed that the care-co-ordinators can have 2–3 people on their individual caseloads at any one time. This means 12 (30/2.5) clinicians will be needed for this function.

Thus a total of 18 staff are needed for assessment and key worker functions. It is assumed that this will be provided by CPNs and social workers and the remainder of the team will support these core staff (see Box 11).

Fewer additional workers have been placed in these teams to reflect the shorter-term contact that they have with patients.

Box 11: WTE staff required for a total population of 250,000 – CRTs	
Consultant psychiatrists	1
Other medical staff	1
Clinical psychologists	1
Team leaders	1
CPNs	14
Social workers	4
Pharmacists	0.5
Pharmacy technicians	0.3
Support workers	See section on support workers (p35)
Admin. staff	1
Total	**23.8**

This means a total of 5,755 staff are required for 207 CRTs for England by 2010.

How does this compare to other estimates?

The NHS Plan proposed 335 dedicated teams across England by the end of 2004. In 2003 there were 125 Crisis Resolution Teams in England (Glover *et al.*, 2004), rising to 168 by March 2004 (Department of Health, 2004a). In Spring 2006 there were 268 teams (one per 119,796 adult population) with 4,862 staff (4,322 care staff) (Centre for Public Mental Health, Durham University, 2006). Whilst the number of teams is rising there is a shortfall in the staff required.

Early intervention in psychosis teams (EITs)

Early intervention teams (EITs) were introduced to offer tailored care and support to people aged between 14 and 35 experiencing their first episode of psychosis. Their aim is to identify young people who are developing a severe mental health condition and to provide them with a service that is appropriate to their age group and personal situation.

The MHPIG (Department of Health, 2001a) gives figures for new users and total caseloads for teams covering one million total population. It estimates that there will be 150 new cases per year and that each will see the service for three years. This gives a total caseload of approximately 450. The PIG suggests dividing the service into a number of teams (three or four), each managing a caseload of 30 to 50 new cases per year and 120 to 150 in total. The suggested staffing levels cover a team with a caseload of 120 to 150. They include a total of 10 WTE care co-ordinators (including team leader) with a service user to care co-ordinator ratio of 15 to 1. It also recommends that the team includes 0.5 WTE adult consultant psychiatrists, 1.0 WTE non-career grade psychiatrist and 0.1 WTE child and adolescent (CAMHS) consultant psychiatrists.

The number of new cases of psychosis that occur each year is about 38 per 250,000, which is identical to that quoted in the PIG. The overall PIG figures will therefore be used to calculate the staffing numbers: 135 cases per team with caseload per care co-ordinator of 10 (13.5 care co-ordinators). The figures are shown in Box 12.

Additional workers have been placed in these teams. The employment lead may be of particular significance given the importance of getting this group of users into meaningful occupation. The role could be carried out by any mental health professional with the appropriate skills and experience, but may be suitable for those with an occupational therapy background.

The national requirement for 2010 is 207 teams and 4,844 staff.

Box 12: WTE staff required for a total population of 250,000 – Early intervention teams (EITs)	
Consultant psychiatrists (adult)	0.5
Consultant psychiatrists (CAMHS)	0.1
Other medical staff	1
Clinical psychologists	1
Team leaders	1 } Total
CPNs	9 } care
Social workers	2 } co-ordinators
OTs	1.5 } = 13.5
OT assistants	1
Pharmacists	0.5
Pharmacy technicians	0.3
Psychology technicians	0.5
Dual diagnosis workers	1
Employment leads	1
Employment specialists	1
Support workers	See section on support workers (p35)
Admin. staff	2
Total	**23.4**

How does this compare to other estimates?

1. The NHS Plan set a target of 50 early intervention teams by the end of 2004. In 2003 there were 36 early intervention teams in England (Glover *et al.*, 2004). By the time of the five-year NSF-MH review (Department of Health, 2004a) there were 41 teams and the review acknowledged that the formation of these teams lagged behind that of the other modernisation teams. The teams were smaller than planned, employing a total of 174 staff. In Spring 2006 the Durham AMH mapping data reported 128 teams (one per 119,796 adult population) with 932 care staff (Centre for Public Mental Health, Durham University, 2006). The numbers of teams and staff are rising but lag behind the numbers required.

2. Lambeth Early Onset (LEO) in south London. This is a well-staffed team with a good service that serves an area with a rate of onset of first episodes of psychosis of around 40/100,000. LEO takes all referrals of people aged 16–35 with a possible or definite psychosis from Lambeth (pop 265,000 adults). The team sees approximately 90 new cases per year. The LEO service consists of two teams. An assessment team (LEO-CAT) is made up of 7.5 WTE staff. It works with GPs, A&E

departments and other agencies, does initial assessments and initiates treatment before handing over to the LEO community team. The LEO community team consists of 12.7 WTE staff and provides continuing care and supervision for 2 years. The total staffing is thus 20.2 WTE.

The proposed early intervention teams have the potential to improve the services for young people with psychoses significantly and have a preventative function. Sustained investment and recruitment are required to increase the number of teams with adequate numbers of suitably trained staff.

Support services

Support workers

The evidence on which to base the use of support workers comes mainly from user satisfaction studies and opinions of mental health workers and managers (Mental Aftercare Association, 2002; Department of Health 2001b; Murray *et al.*, 1997) and is supported by DH policy (Department of Health, 2003a). The Workforce Action Team (WAT) report (Department of Health, 2001b) considered the non-professionally affiliated workforce in mental health services and came up with the idea of the support, time and recovery (STR) worker who they considered would make up a largely new staff group that should be paid at a rate commensurate with their skills, experience and responsibilities. They estimated that about 10,000 STR workers would be required for England.

The Policy Implementation Guide on STR workers (Department of Health, 2003a) defined the STR worker as "*...someone who works as part of a team which provides mental health services and focuses on the needs of service users, working across boundaries of care, organisation and role*", "*They will provide Support, give Time to the service users and thus promote their Recovery*". They may be employed by any employer in the NHS or social care field, including the private and voluntary sector.

There is already a cadre of support workers in mental health services, employed across the public and voluntary sectors, some of whom have a role similar to that envisaged for the STR workers. The STR PIG suggests that, over time, the existing community support workers may be assimilated into the STR role (Department of Health, 2003a).

We have based our overall calculations on the same figures as used in the WAT report. i.e. the number of people with severe and enduring mental illness reported in Box 8. The numbers proposed for each team are based on the figures given in the WAT report for STR workers (Department of Health, 2001b). The WAT report assumed that one third of service users would require a STR worker and that each STR worker could have a caseload of 10 people, giving a need for 10,000 STR workers for England. This means that 50 STR workers are required for a total population of 250,000. These workers could be used in a number of ways in this catchment area, including being divided between the CMHTs, AOTs, CRTs and early onset services in proportions roughly commensurate with the caseload sizes of the teams. The role of these workers is set out in the relevant PIG (Department of Health, 2003a).

The Durham AMH mapping data for Spring 2006 reported that there were 1,958 STR workers employed in England, 1001 gateway workers and 160 BME workers (Centre for Public Mental Health, Durham University, 2006).

Other services

In addition to the core health and social services teams, community-based support services will also be required. They may include:

1. Advice and information services. These already exist at the national level, e.g. NHS Direct, Samaritans. It would also be expected that all teams would have information about their local services available for users and carers.
2. Advocacy services.
3. Befriending and voluntary schemes.
4. Self-help and mutual aid groups.
5. Service user groups.

These types of service are often run locally by the voluntary sector and may vary locally. In view of this the costs of these services may often not directly fall on the health and social services. For example, the Citizens Advice Bureau (CAB) provides free and independent advice in 751 GP surgeries and health centres, 62 general hospitals, 75 psychiatric hospitals and 165 mental health clinics (Citizens Advice Bureau, 2005). In addition, since 2003 the Department of Health has funded CAB to provide Independent Complaints Advocacy Service (ICAS) services in six of nine health regions in England and there are 116 ICAS specialists based in 32 bureaux. This funding has been extended to 2006. The CAB runs advice projects specifically for people with mental health problems in over 100 Bureaux advising on debt, housing, employment and benefit entitlements (Citizens Advice Bureau, 2005). These schemes are in line with the Public Health White Paper *Choosing Health* (Department of Health, 2004h) and may make contributions to four key themes of the strategy: supporting families, mothers and children; engaging communities and individuals; preventing illness and providing effective treatment and care; and addressing the underlying determinants of health.

5 Standards 4 & 5
Inpatient services

What type of service?

Community services must be backed up by good-quality acute inpatient services. It is assumed that they must provide places for asylum, for crisis management and for therapeutic activity. They should be supported by a range of residential accommodation and rehabilitation facilities.

For the inpatient and residential units it has been assumed that:

1. Staffing levels on wards should reflect the additional staff required to improve care and therapeutic activity requirements in these residential units. For example the acute inpatient units should be able to provide increased amounts of psychosocial care and activities as well as manage crises safely and securely. The rehabilitation units should provide active rehabilitation and link to specialist and community facilities.
2. Psychiatric intensive care units (PICUs) will be required and the size of a PICU is eight beds.
3. Staffing should be made up of a mixture of professions and of qualified and non-qualified staff.

Epidemiological base

The types of inpatient services and numbers of beds have been based on figures from the National Beds Inquiry (Department of Health, 2000c). As part of its remit the Inquiry examined the need for inpatient and residential care for those with mental health problems. It provided estimates for the numbers of beds required for a range of facilities, including acute and residential units. It did not give estimates for the staff that would be required for these units. The estimates are shown in Box 13 and compared to current estimates.

Box 13: National Beds Inquiry projections for inpatient and residential care

	2005/06	2010/11	2003 estimated provision (from Durham Mapping report, 2004 unless stated)*
	Number of places	*Number of places*	*Number of places*
High secure	994	816	Approx 900[1]
Medium secure and long-term secure	2,592	2,543	4,433[2]
PICU	1,429	1,583	812 PICU + 751 low secure, high dependency
Acute inpatient	16,097	15,934	20,319
NHS long-stay	1,761	0	2,701 residential rehabilitation beds
24-hour staffed beds	4,100	5,853	1,492 NHS 24-hour nurse staffed care + 2,719 residential care homes
High staffed hostel	15,608	14,873	6,254 registered care homes[3]
Day-staffed hostel	9,635	7,532	1,076 staffed group homes
Unstaffed group homes	5,661	7,461	943 unstaffed group homes + 13,462 supported housing places

* (Glover *et al.*, 2004)

1 From Fender (2004)
2 Laing and Buisson (2006)
3 The Durham Mapping report suggested that these figures may be unreliable as older adult places may be included (Glover *et al.*, 2004).

The projections from the National Beds Inquiry for 2010–2011 have been used in most cases to calculate the staffing required. Two types of inpatient service are absent from the National Beds Inquiry projections:

1. **Rehabilitation units.** We believe that the estimates for inpatient rehabilitation may be unrealistic as it is difficult to foresee no need for rehabilitation inpatient units for the groups of people with severe and enduring mental health problems. We have thus used what we believe is a reasonable estimate of 10 beds per 250,000 population.

2. **Low secure units.** The Inquiry did not include these units which are included in the Mental Health Policy Implementation Guide on Psychiatric Intensive Care and Low Secure Environments (Department of Health, 2002d). The units operate along the principles of rehabilitation for people who require the provision of security (Department of Health, 2002d; page 4). A reasonable estimate for the provision of low secure beds is 10 per 250,000.

The inpatient provision for forensic services is discussed in Chapter 7.

The calculations for each type of unit will be taken in turn.

Acute inpatient units

There is no generally accepted formula for calculating the nursing establishment and associated grade mix for acute inpatient units (e.g. Warr, 1995; Buchan & Dal Poz, 2002).

Several approaches exist (Buchan *et al.*, 2000), but the calculations here use the professional judgment approach (Cox, 2004). This approach asks professionals to assess ward activity and review available information in order to reach a consensus judgment concerning the number of nurses required to effectively manage a ward. The estimates made here assume that the bed numbers will decline but the people who are admitted will be more acutely ill and require high levels of nursing. In addition the ward will function as a therapeutic environment and nursing and other staff will require time to undertake these necessary activities.

Our calculation assumes that nurses on a 20-bed unit will work in shifts of six early, six late and four on nights. This will require a complement of 25 nurses to cover the ward for a seven day period. On top of this, allowance needs to be made for absences which include:

Paid leave	17.0% (reflecting *Agenda for Change* [Department of Health, 1998e] adjustments).
Training	4.1% (including professional development, supervision and appraisal)
Sickness	5.0% (based on a target of 13 days per year)
Practice governance	2.3% (including research and audit work)

This gives a total increase of 28.4% on the basic staffing level. Thus for a 20-bedded ward the total number of nurses required is 25 plus 28.4% i.e. 32.1 staff.

Our calculation also assumes that:

- The ward manager should be full-time and supernumerary.
- The modern matron role (Department of Health, 2000a) is additional to the ward manager role.
- There are two deputy ward managers who focus on practice development, leadership and management support, but are not supernumerary.
- The ratio of qualified to unqualified is set at 70:30, but need not be rigid and should reflect local conditions and priorities. Thus for a 20-bedded ward 22.5 qualified and 10.6 unqualified staff are required.

The use of supernumerary ward managers, deputy ward managers and the ratio of 70:30 qualified to unqualified staff are assumed for each of the hospital units below.

Psychiatric intensive care units (PICUs)

For an eight-bedded PICU it is assumed that:

1. Five staff are required to cover the early and late shifts, while four are needed for the night shifts. This means that 21 nurses are required to cover over 7 days.
2. The same 28.4% addition as for acute units is required, taking the total to 26.9 staff.
3. The ratio of qualified to unqualified is 70:30 (18.8 qualified and 8.1 unqualified).

Low secure units

For a ten-bedded low secure unit it is assumed that:

1. Four staff are required to cover the early and late shifts, with three covering the night shifts. This means that 17 nurses are required to cover for 7 days.
2. The same 28.4% addition as for acute units is required – 21.8 staff required.
3. The ratio of qualified to unqualified is 70:30 (15.26 qualified and 6.54 unqualified).

Rehabilitation ward

For a ten-bedded rehabilitation ward it is assumed that:

1. Four staff are required to cover the early and late shifts, with two covering the night shifts. This means that 15 nurses are required to cover for seven days.
2. The same 28.4% addition as for acute units is required – 19.26 staff required.
3. The ratio of qualified to unqualified is 70:30 (13.5 qualified and 5.76 unqualified).

The rehabilitation ward will be run as part of the district specialist rehabilitation services. Consultant medical staff will cover both the inpatient and community rehabilitation services. The community rehabilitation team will cover all the hostel accommodation in the 250,000 population (see later).

24-hour hostel accommodation

For a ten-bedded 24-hour hostel it is assumed that:

1. Three staff are required to cover the early and late shifts and two at night. Twelve nurses are thus required to cover for 7 days.
2. The same 28.4% addition as for acute units is required – 15.4 staff required.
3. The ratio of qualified to unqualified is 70:30 (10.78 qualified and 4.62 unqualified).

Other hostel accommodation

The other staffed hostels will need one member of staff for each bed.

The staff will all be support workers and may be managed by a voluntary sector organisation. This type of accommodation may also be considered under the Supporting People strategy (Office of Deputy Prime Minister, 2004)

These nursing estimates have been combined with estimates for other staff. The full staffing estimates for these inpatient and residential units are shown in Box 14.

Additional staff for inpatient units

It is assumed that medical and nursing staff are required for all inpatient units. Other staff have been added using the following rationales:

1. **Need to improve medicines management and the physical care for patients.**

   Pharmacists – The basis for their inclusion is the same as for the community units. The use of pharmacists as part of the inpatient multidisciplinary team is specifically mentioned in the Policy Implementation Guide on Psychiatric Intensive Care and Low Secure Environments (Department of Health, 2002d).

   Dieticians – Physical disorders are common among people with psychiatric disorders and are often inadequately detected and managed, as are their dietary inadequacies. The Policy Implementation Guide on Acute Inpatient Care Provision (Department of Health, 2002b) highlights that physical care and dietary requirements are often neglected. It also highlights that the need for greater access and regular input to the inpatient ward, and its organisation and activities by dieticians, should be clearly defined and deliverable. Medical and nursing staff need to refer people with complex therapeutic dietary requirements such as in coeliac disease, newly diagnosed and unstable diabetes, obesity, hyperlipidaemia, malnutrition and food refusal.

   The NSF for Diabetes (Department of Health, 2001e) states that everyone admitted to hospital for whatever reason should access dietary information and support. In addition, as part of the better hospital food programme, dieticians are expected to check hospital menus to ensure all nutritional requirements can be met, and inpatients are entitled to access a dietician when prescribed a special diet. (http://195.92.246.148/nhsestates/better_hospital_food/bhf_content/introduction/home.asp; Department of Health, 2004h; 2004i). People on inpatient wards need access to a healthy diet appropriate to their needs. In an inpatient setting many people omit breakfast and/or other meals, preferring to snack on refined carbohydrates with a high saturated fat content thus contributing to the weight gain associated with many medications.

2. **To increase the available therapies and activities.**

   To address this, occupational therapists, clinical psychologist and creative therapists have been added to the sessional input into inpatient units.

3. **To increase the social care component of inpatient units**

   Dedicated social workers have been added to several of the units. They will also provide input relating to the Mental Health Act. Input from workers providing benefit and employment advice and support may be provided by the workers in the community teams. STR workers from the staff pool described in Chapter 4 may also be designated to have input into the inpatient and other residential units.

Box 14: Projected number of residential places for an illustrative total population of 250,000 in year 2010 and the associated staff

Facility	Beds	Psychiatrists				Clinical psychologists		Nurses			Occupational therapists			Therapists		Social workers	Pharmacists		Dieticians	Support workers
	National Beds Inquiry provision by 2010–11	Cons	SpR	SHO	Staff grade	Qualified	Techn-ician	Ward manager	Regis-tered	Health-care assist-ants	Exper-ienced	Basic grade	Techn-ical Instruc-tor	Psycho thera-pist	Art, Music, Drama		Quali-fied	Techn-ician		
Medium secure[1]	21	1.5	0.75	1.5	0.75	1.5	1.5	1.5	28.2	12.2	1.5	1.5	1.5	0.75		1.5	0.45	0.15	0.45	
PICU/ Local secure	8	1.0	0.2	1.0		0.4	0.4	1.0	18.8	8.1	0.8						0.3	0.1	0.1	
Low secure[2]	10	1.0	0.2	1.0		0.5	0.5	1.0	15.26	6.54	1.0		1.0		0.2	0.5	0.3	0.1	0.3	
Acute hospital	80	4.0	2.0	4.0	2.0	4.0	4.0	4.0 + 1.0 Modern Matron	89.9	38.5	4.0	4.0	2.0	0.5	1.0	4.0	1.0	1.0	1	
Rehabili-tation[2]	10	1.0	1.0		1.0	1.0	1.0	1.0	13.5	5.76	1.0		1.0			0.5	0.3	0.1	0.3	
24-hr staffed	30							3.0	27.0	11.52										
High staffed hostel	75																			75 (+3 mgrs)
Day staffed hostel	38																			38 (+2 mgrs)
Unstaffed group homes	38																			
Total		**8.5**	**4.15**	**7.5**	**3.75**	**7.4**	**7.4**	**11.5+1**	**192.66**	**82.62**	**8.3**	**5.5**	**5.5**	**1.25**	**1.2**	**6.5**	**2.35**	**1.45**	**2.15**	**113.0**

1 Number of MSU beds taken from Laing and Buisson (2006)
2 NHS Inpatient Rehabilitation units and Low Secure Units were not included in the National Beds Inquiry projects for 2010/2011.

Cons = consultant SpR = specialist registrar SHO = senior house officer

6 Standards 4 & 5 Day care and employment schemes

What type of service?

There is no currently widely accepted model for day care, but recent guidance for commissioners of mental health services on day services for working-age adults with mental health problems emphasises the need to refocus present services into community resources that promote social inclusion (Department of Health, 2006a). This is consistent with other policy initiatives including the NSF-MH (Department of Health, 1999), Social Exclusion report (Social Exclusion Unit, 2004), Choosing Health White Paper (Department of Health, 2004h), the Adult Social Care Green Paper (Department of Health, 2005g) and the Health, Work and Well-being strategy (HM Government, 2005a). The guidance outlines principles for re-focusing day services which include:

- Promoting recovery
- A focus on community participation
- Reducing social isolation
- Offering opportunities for people with mental health problems to provide support to each other and to run their own services
- Maximising choice and self-determination
- Meeting the needs of diverse groups
- Ensuring that services are accessible to people who are more seriously disabled by their mental health problems
- Involving users and carers
- Increasing diversity of provision
- Improving cross-sector working.

It views the functions of day services as being to:

- Provide opportunities for social contact and support.
- Support people to retain existing social roles, relationships and existing social and leisure activities that they value.
- Support people to access new roles, relationships and maintain social and leisure activities of their choosing.
- Provide opportunities for people with mental health problems to run their own services.

An additional document on commissioning women-only day services (Department of Health, 2006b) outlines the types of services required for women. This builds on the commitment made in the NHS Plan (Department of Health, 2000a) for the provision of a women-only day centre for every health authority by 2004. The types of services envisaged include:

- Drop-in facilities
- Childcare support
- Parenting support
- Educational programmes
- Therapeutic interventions and activities
- Befriending schemes
- Crisis support
- Help lines
- Information facilities.

The actual structure and details of the future day services are not specified in the guidance, nor are the staffing needs. It emphasises the utilisation of staff that fit with the ten essential shared capabilities for mental health practice (Department of Health, 2004k).

The commissioning guidance forms the basis of the staffing requirements and costs outlined here. It is already known that many parts of the country experience a dearth of day provision and have a very narrow provision of services. Yet day care run by the voluntary sector can be creative and acceptable to service users. Recent Rethink reports (Rethink, 2004; 2005) highlighted the need for access to services of many people with enduring mental health problems who may have many unmet needs and may benefit from stable day services.

The principles of the services considered here are that:

- There should be a spectrum of such services, including appropriate day services, for example for women and BME groups.
- Services may be flexible in their referral criteria and times of opening. Some may be open five days per week and between 9.00–5.00, whilst others may operate extended hours or weekend opening.
- They should support the other mental health teams and inpatient services in the area.
- They are generally not directly run by the NHS, but by social services or the independent sector.
- The local NHS mental health trust should help support the services through some form of umbrella body, through which day care activity is co-ordinated. This may include securing agreement about referral so that one referral form covers all the day care or that service users can attend sessions at more than one centre. This gives more choice and flexibility.
- Links should also be made to non-mental health provision such as leisure services.

For vocational services a similar spectrum and flexibility of service is required which provides links with educational and training facilities. In addition, there should be links with volunteer organisations such as the local volunteer bureau, time banks and the Capital Volunteering Scheme. The spectrum of such services could include: supported employment (there is an evidence base for these), social firms, transitional employment schemes and sheltered employment. These services may not be devoted only to those with mental health conditions and are paid for by block contracts or by individual payments.

It is assumed that, in the service proposed, there may be little use for NHS day hospitals as many of these may be replaced by the new community teams. Day centres and drop-in services can cater for a wider group of users and for BME groups and women. Leisure and educational services may be provided by local authorities and some link workers may be added to assist with these.

Epidemiological base

It is assumed that the day care and employment services will cater for over half of the 430 people on enhanced CPA for a population of 250,000 at any one time. There will be an additional group of people with long-term problems who are not on CPA and will also require some day service contact. Rethink (2004; 2005) estimated that 50,000 people had been in contact with services over a long period of time, their needs had stabilised but their quality of life, and that of their carers, remained poor.

To estimate the staff required for meaningful daytime activity, the current provision in one London borough, which may be considered as an example of good practice, has been used as a guide. The day services cover a mixed inner city population of 250,000 and include no NHS provision. They offer a range of services and some operate after 5.00 pm and at weekends. One centre is for African and Caribbean people. At present the services have a total of 36 staff. There are no women-only day services in the borough and staffing estimates for this have been added to the overall provision.

To this staffing should be added six 'bridge builders': workers who will offer assistance to users to provide links with other agencies (e.g. employment, voluntary work, education and leisure) in the local community.

Box 15 shows the number of day staff required for a total 250,000 population.

Box 15: WTE staff required for a total population of 250,000 – Day units	
OTs	3.0
Managers	5.0
Deputy managers	5.0
Senior project workers	8.0
Other project workers	20.0
Admin workers	5.0
Bridge builders	6.0
Total	**52**

Vocational services

It is known that many people with severe mental health problems are economically inactive (Social Exclusion Unit, 2004) and that many people with mental health problems are on incapacity benefit (HM Government, 2005b). Present government policy addresses the need to decrease the numbers of people with mental health problems who are on incapacity benefit and to increase the employment rate of this group (HM Government, 2006).

Recent guidance on vocational services for people with severe mental health problems published jointly by the Departments of Health and Work and Pensions (Department of Health/Department for Work and Pensions, 2006) attempts to provide commissioners of mental health services with a framework to commission evidence-based vocational services and tools to monitor effectiveness.

This is consistent with action points detailed in the Social Exclusion report (Social Exclusion Unit, 2004) and the Choosing Health White Paper (Department of Health, 2004h). It is also consistent with the NSF-MH, the Framework for Vocational Rehabilitation (Department for Work and Pensions, 2004) and the strategy for health and well-being in working-age people (HM Government, 2005a).

The Vocational Guidance (Department of Health/Department for Work and Pensions, 2006) lists five key elements to a comprehensive range of vocational services for people with severe mental health problems:

1. Clinical support leads within secondary services. These are seen as mental health professionals within each team, who take a clinical perspective on vocational rehabilitation. They offer advice and guidance on vocational matters to other team members and provide brief interventions that help clients to achieve their vocational preferences and choice.

2. Employment specialists integrated within clinical teams (including CMHTs, the modernisation teams and rehabilitation teams). These people do not necessarily require a health or social services background. Their role is to identify and assess clients' vocational needs, help them to gain and retain employment, education and voluntary work and provide continuing support.

3. Public services as exemplar employers.

4. Supported work opportunities. Support may be offered to employees while they are in mainstream employment by a third-party provider. For those people who would benefit from a specially constructed workplace, social enterprises and firms may be useful options.

5. Local partnership arrangements between specialist and mainstream providers with appropriate commissioner input.

The clinical support leads and employment specialists have been included in the staffing estimates for the community teams (see earlier). The supported schemes may be run by independent sector organisations. Other aspects are matters for the working of organisations and not dependent on additional staff.

How does this compare to other estimates?

In 2003 the services reported in England (Glover *et al.*, 2004) were:

264 NHS day services across
711 day centres or resource centres
183 CMHT day centre services
397 drop-in services
150 sheltered employment services
289 training and education services
238 supported employment services

In spring 2006 there were 2,221 staff in day care/resource centres, 615 staff in drop-in centres and 727 staff in employment and training services (Centre for Public Mental Health, Durham University, 2006). This gives a total of 3,563 staff which can be compared to the staff requirement of 10,756 estimated from Box 15, a third of the required level.

It is not certain how many different types of work scheme operate in England. Some surveys estimate that there are at least 135 organisations offering sheltered employment, 77 providing open employment and about 50 social firms (Crowther *et al.*, 2001; Grove & Durie, 1999). A survey in the northwest of England found high variation in provision and a poor relationship between the schemes identified and the needs of the areas in which they operated (Crowther & Marshall, 2001).

Current provision suggests that there is a need to develop clearer models and a policy on day care and vocational services that equates with developments in social inclusion.

7 Standards 4 & 5
Forensic services

Forensic services deal with people at the interface of law and mental health services. They are concerned with the assessment, treatment and clinical management of mentally disordered people who have committed grave offences (or are deemed capable of committing grave offences). These services have mainly been based in inpatient units, the high secure units (Broadmoor, Ashworth and Rampton) and in medium secure units which offer shorter-term assessment and treatment. There has been less emphasis on community-based forensic services, although this is changing.

Forensic service inpatient beds

There is an insufficient understanding of the capacity required for forensic beds over the next decade. The Department of Health has commissioned an independent report on requirements for medium and high secure services, but this is not yet in the public domain. It seems unlikely that there will be a reduction in the number of beds required and the estimates given in the National Beds Inquiry may prove to be too low.

One difficulty in calculating the high and medium secure bed requirements is that forensic services are essentially capacity based. Figures on the prison populations suggest a high level of unmet need for which forensic services have inadequate capacity. Future developments will bring additional pressures on forensic services. These include the implications of the amended Mental Health Act; the Criminal Justice Act 2003 in which sentences aimed to protect the public will be based on actuarial assessments of risk; the development of dangerous and severe personality disorder (DSPD) services; the impact of multi-agency public protection arrangements; and the creation of mental health teams for prisons (Department of Health/HM Prison Service, 2001).

High secure beds

Currently, high secure beds are based in the three special hospitals (Broadmoor, Rampton and Ashworth). The number of people resident in the three hospitals has reduced since 1985 from a peak of 1,750 to 1,300 at the end of 1999 when a survey was carried out to examine the beds in high secure hospitals (Fender, 2004). Between 2000 and 2004 the Accelerated Discharge Programme (ADP) led to the redistribution of 400 patients to medium secure units, thus further lowering the number of residents.

The present plans are to keep each secure hospital and to have each take patients from specific parts of England and Wales. All women will be based at Rampton as will patients with learning difficulties and those who are deaf. New DSPD units will be based at Broadmoor and Rampton. Fender (2004) gave projections for 2010 of:

Ashworth – about 210 beds required
Broadmoor – about 257 beds required
Rampton – about 353 beds required

These figures are in agreement with the 820 beds projected by the National Beds Inquiry for 2010/2011 and have been used to calculate staffing requirements. Our staff numbers per bed have been based on those for medium secure units (MSUs) but increased in line with the higher unit costs for high secure provision.

Medium secure beds

Currently there are 4,433 medium secure beds in England (21 per 250,000 population): 2,888 in the NHS and 1,545 in the independent sector (Laing & Buisson, 2006).

The National Beds Inquiry suggested 13 per 250,000 population (total of 2,543 projected for 2010/2011). This may now be regarded as an under-estimate and may need to be revised in the future. In view of this the current number of 4,433 beds (21 per 250,000) has been used in the staffing calculations for MSUs in this report (see Box 14)

For 21 beds in a medium secure unit it is assumed that:

1. The number of staff required to cover the early, late and night shifts for a 14-bedded unit are the same as for an eight-bedded PICU (thus for a 21-bedded unit the figures are proportionate and increased by a factor of 1.5): 7.5 for early and late shifts and six at night. 31.5 nurses are required to cover for 7 days.
2. The same 28.4% addition of staff is required, as in acute units – 40.4 staff required.
3. The ratio of qualified to unqualified is 70:30 (28.2 qualified and 12.2 unqualified).

See Box 14 for the actual staffing of MSUs.

Community forensic teams

There may be some parallel here with general adult community schemes, but these teams are presently in their infancy and there is no guidance as to their structure and function. There is a need to consider the community management of offenders and those discharged from secure services and these teams may cover these tasks. Components of such a service may include:

- Consultation/liaison with local CMHTs to advise on risk and criminal justice matters, including advice on patients with complex needs involving risk and/or offending.
- Management of a small caseload of high risk individuals in the community and patients on restriction orders with complex needs.
- Providing a resource to multi-agency public protection arrangements (MAPPA) in the area.
- Consultation/liaison to probation and other agencies within the national offender management system.
- Overseeing court liaison and court diversion arrangements.

The actual number of people requiring support from this team is not known, but based on teams operating in south London the desirable staffing for an area of 250,000 total population might be that shown in Box 16.

Box 16: WTE staff required for a total population of 250,000 – Community forensic teams	
Consultant psychiatrist	1
Specialist registrar (SpR)	1
Clinical psychologist	1
CPNs	5
Social workers	3
Administrator/secretary	1
Total	**12**

There are no current data indicating how many of these teams exist in England, but anecdotal evidence suggests there are few.

Prison in-reach services

The NSF-MH applies to all working-age adults, including prisoners. The Department of Health and Prison Service set out their strategy for modernising mental health services in prisons in December 2001 (Department of Health/HM Prison Service, 2001). The aim was to provide a range of services available to prisoners over the forthcoming three to five years, in line with the NSF-MH and the NHS Plan.

What type of service?

There are three major groups at which services should be aimed: those with mental disorders, those with substance abuse and those with learning difficulties.

Two types of team are required:

1. The equivalent of CMHTs for prisons (these may also incorporate a dedicated member of a learning disability service within the team).
2. Dedicated substance misuse teams. These teams could consist of addiction nurses and specially trained prison staff, with input from GPs. They may link with similar workers, for example CARAT (care, assessment, rehabilitation and throughcare) and PASRO (prisoners addressing substance related offending) workers. They could offer detoxification, drug counselling, methadone maintenance and other pharmacological treatment and encourage seamless throughcare.

Epidemiological base

The distribution and prevalence of mental health problems in prisons differ substantially from those in the general population and people with mental health problems are significantly over-represented in the prison population. Multiple diagnoses are common. The Singleton *et al.* (1998) study found that nine out of ten prisoners met their criteria for at least one mental health diagnosis, most of whom had more than one.

There are 139 prisons in England and Wales. About 140,000 people pass through English and Welsh prisons in any one year. At the end of September 2005 there are approximately 77,000 people in prison (HM Prison Service, 2005) and that figure is projected to rise to 91,500 by 2010 (Home Office, 2005).

In an average male prison (for example Brixton with 800 prisoners) the ONS study (Singleton *et al.*, 1998) would suggest that up to 720 prisoners will have mental health symptoms meeting a research definition for a mental disorder including:

- 48 with schizophrenia
- 320 with depression, anxiety and related conditions
- 272 dependent on drugs
- 512 with personality disorder.

Self-harm and completed suicide are also present at a substantially higher level than in the general population.

There is a very high use of drugs and alcohol among prisoners (Borrill *et al.*, 2003; Litiano & Ramsey, 2003; Bullock, 2003). Before imprisonment:

- About half of prisoners have used cocaine or heroin recently.
- 82% of heroin users and 37% of crack cocaine users were consuming it every day.
- Over 60% used cannabis and 40% amphetamine.
- 66% of heroin users were also consuming crack cocaine.
- 54% of prisoners were using at least one type of illegal drug daily before imprisonment.
- About 50% give evidence of moderate or severe dependence.
- Severe dependence is found more frequently in women.
- About 30% had "severe alcohol problems" (Litiano & Ramsey, 2003; Bullock, 2003).

Drug withdrawal on admission may lead to self-harm. 11% of suicides occur during the first 24 hours in prison, 33% in the first week and 47% in the first month. Of these, 62% of these are problematic drug users (HM Prison Service, 2001).

While in prison, the frequency of drug misuse in general is much less than outside prison, but 54% of prisoners use cannabis, 27% heroin and 15% illicitly obtained tranquillisers. Use of other drugs is less common, for example 7% still use cocaine, 3% on a daily basis (Singleton *et al.*, 1998), while 44% of those using drugs before imprisonment abstain while in prison. Yet about 25% of those who have ever used heroin used it for the first time while in prison (Bullock, 2003).

There are wide variations in the estimates on the number of offenders with learning difficulties in prisons. Murphy *et al.* (1995) surveyed 157 male prisoners in HM Prison Belmarsh and found that 33 responded that they had a learning difficulty or had attended special school.

Service requirements

A report on prison psychiatry from the Royal College of Psychiatrists (2005) recommended that the number of consultant psychiatrist posts required depends on the size and nature of the prison:

Category B local remand prison of 500 places (Category B are prisoners who do not require maximum security, but for whom escape needs to be made difficult):

0.5 WTE consultant (general adult or forensic)
0.5 WTE non-consultant grade.
Plus 0.2 WTE addiction specialist sessions and
Psychotherapy input – 3 sessions

Category A local remand prison of 500 places (Category A are prisoners whose escape would be highly dangerous to the public or national security):

0.75 WTE consultant (general adult or forensic)
0.5 WTE non consultant grade.
Plus 0.2 WTE addiction specialist sessions and
Psychotherapy input – 3 sessions.

Category B dispersal prison of 500 places
0.5 WTE (forensic or forensic rehabilitation)
0.5 WTE non consultant grade and
Psychotherapy input – 3 sessions.

Category C and D dispersal prison (Category C are prisoners who cannot be trusted in open conditions but who are unlikely to try to escape; Category D are prisoners who are trusted enough to wander freely but must show up for daily roll calls).

These are unlikely to require a full psychiatric team so perhaps 0.3 WTE per 500 places but with some access to specialist services through a mental health trust.

The staffing required for teams for a hypothetical category B prison of 550 inmates is shown in Box 17.

Box 17: WTE staff required for a hypothetical category B prison of 550 inmates

CMHT staff	WTE
Consultant psychiatrist	0.5
Consultant psychotherapist	0.3
Staff grade doctor	0.5
Clinical psychologist	0.5
CPNs (including 1 LD* trained)	3
OT	1
OT helpers	2
Technical instructors	1.2
Social worker or probation officer	0.5
Counsellor	0.5
Creative therapist	0.5
Speech and language therapist	0.5
Total	**11.0**
Substance misuse team staff	**WTE**
Addiction specialist	0.2
CPNs	3
Total	**3.2**

*LD = learning disability

If there are 58 Category A and B remand and dispersal prisons in England with approximately 32,395 places then, assuming that the numbers of staff above are required for 550 inmates, 648 CMHT staff and 188 substance misuse staff are needed for these services. There are 43 category C and open prisons with approximately 20,935 places; if 0.3 consultant psychiatrists are required for 500 places then 13 additional consultant psychiatrists are required. The figures for the prisons are taken from HM Prison Service (2005).

8 Standards 4 & 5
Sub-speciality services

The main specialist adult services outlined in this document will require additional support for specific groups of service users. These sub-speciality services include general hospital liaison services, perinatal services, services for people with eating disorders and personality disorders and services for deaf people. These services may cover populations in excess of 250,000.

1. Liaison psychiatry services

Services required

These are for the provision of general services to an entire acute hospital, with possibly some sessional input into specific units, for example oncology units, although additional funding may be needed for these.

Epidemiological base

The figures for liaison services have been taken from the Royal College of Psychiatrists/Royal College of Physicians (2003) Report. The figures are based on:

1. Estimates of likely demand (from House and Hodgson, 1994).
2. A district general hospital of 600 beds in a catchment area of 250,000.
3. Provision of general services to the entire hospital, with some liaison with specialist units.
4. For a teaching hospital in an inner city area, with many specialist and tertiary centres – extra staff may be required, e.g. two full-time consultants.

Estimated workload	**Annual rate of patients seen**
Deliberate self-harm (DSH)	500
A&E episodes	200
Ward referrals	200
Outpatient contacts	
New	100–150
Follow-up	500
Specific liaison with one or two units	100

The staffing required is shown in Box 18.

Box 18: WTE staff required for a total population of 250,000 – General hospital liaison services	
Consultant	1.0
Specialist registrar (SpR)	1.0
Senior house officer (SHO)	1.0
Liaison nurses	5.0
Clinical or health psychologists	2.0
Secretary	1.0
Total	**11.0**

2. Perinatal services

Services required

These services are targeted at women with significant mental health problems complicating pregnancy and the postpartum year, as well as those women with serious mental health problems who are considering a pregnancy. The types of services, integrated and encompassing both adult (maternal) mental health and (maternity) liaison psychiatry, that are required include:

- A mother and baby unit (either provided locally or on a regional basis).
- Outpatient clinics for both current morbidity in pregnancy and the postpartum period and those at risk of becoming ill.
- Specialist perinatal community mental health team providing both assessment and outreach services.
- Maternity liaison service for both obstetrics and primary maternal health care.
- Parenting skills assessment for those with significant mental illness.
- Day hospital service, particularly for those localities without a mother and baby unit. These services should all be integrated into one perinatal mental health service.

Epidemiological base

Women are at increased risk of developing a serious affective illness following childbirth. Women with pre-existing mental health problems, particularly serious mental illness, are at risk of a relapse or recurrence of their condition during pregnancy and an elevated risk following childbirth. New onset postpartum conditions are predominantly affective but the whole range of psychiatric disorders can present during pregnancy and the postpartum year. The incidence of postpartum psychiatric disorder is usually expressed as that per thousand births (all women delivered) (Royal College of Psychiatrists Report, 2006). The birth rate in the United Kingdom is approximately 11 per 1000 of the population. However the annual birth rate in individual health care localities varies considerably from as low as 6.9 per thousand in some rural areas to as high as 14 per thousand in some inner city areas with large ethnic minority populations. For this reason service planning for a locality or trust area must be predicated upon the annual birth rate rather than the population in general. An average birth rate for a population of 500,000 would be 6,000 live births per year.

Box 19: Rates of mental health disorders in women following delivery

Disorder	Rate per 1,000 births	Number in total population of 500,000
Major depression	100	600
Moderate depression	50	300
Referred to psychiatric services (new episodes of postnatal disorder)	20	120
Referred to psychiatric services in pregnancy	20	120
Admitted with puerperal psychosis	2	12
Admitted with non-psychotic conditions	2	12
Admitted with chronic serious mental illness	2	12

The report on *Perinatal Mental Health Services* (Royal College of Psychiatrists, 2006) gives recommendations for the type and configuration of perinatal services and their organisation into a regional network. Given the rates of admission for perinatal disorders, it will not be possible to have the critical mass of admissions necessary for cost effectiveness and maintenance of knowledge and skills in any but the largest mental health trusts. Mother and baby units should therefore be provided on the basis of larger populations of approximately 1 to 1.5 million of the population. However, the morbidity rates of non-psychotic illnesses are sufficient to justify the provision of a local community perinatal mental health team and maternity liaison service in every locality, in line with official recommendations (Department of Health, 2004l; Confidential Enquiry into Maternal and Child Health, 2004).

The recommended service provision for a delivered population of 14,000 (general population 1.3 million) is:

- A mother and baby inpatient unit – 6 beds.
- Consultant perinatal psychiatrist.
- A multidisciplinary community mental health team.
- Outpatient clinics, a maternity liaison service to both the maternity hospitals and community maternal primary health care.
- A perinatal day hospital, particularly in those localities that do not directly provide a mother and baby unit.

The function of a perinatal mental health service is described in the report on *Perinatal Maternal Mental Health Services* (Royal College of Psychiatrists, 2006). All functions of the perinatal mental health service should be integrated. Those localities that share access to their designated mother and baby unit should work in collaboration with each other. A community perinatal (PN) mental health service will reduce the numbers of admissions and length of stay facilitating alternatives to admission, early discharge and community care.

Box 20: WTE staff required for a delivered population of 14,000 (covering a total population of 1.3 million)	
Medical (work across PN services)	
Consultant psychiatrists	1.5
SpR (specialist registrar)	1.0
SHO (senior house officer)	1.0
Community team	
Nurses (1 nurse manager and 7 G or F grades)	8.0
Social worker (works across PN services)	1.0
Clinical psychologist (works across PN service)	1.0
Mother and baby unit (6 beds)	
Qualified nurses	21
Nursery nurses	7
Day hospital	
Qualified nurses	7
Nursery nurses	7
Admin. support	3

3. Eating disorder services

Services required

These are services directed at people suffering from specific conditions. Eating disorders are most common in young women and the services required are for both adults and adolescents. Adult services will be considered here, but liaison between adolescent services, paediatric services and primary care will be necessary. Two types of service may be required:

1. High intensity treatment team providing outpatient, day patient, inpatient and outreach services.
2. Outpatient treatment team providing outpatient and outreach services.

Epidemiological base

These are taken from the Royal College of Psychiatrists report on *Eating Disorders in the UK* (Royal College of Psychiatrists, 2000). The rates of eating disorders in women are shown in Box 21.

Box 21: Rates of eating disorders in women

Disorder	Incidence	Prevalence	Number in total population of 250,000 (80,822 women aged 16–65 years)
Anorexia nervosa	8.6 per 100,000	0.3%	242
Bulaemia nervosa	12.4 per 100,000	1.0%	808

Box 22 shows the services and staffing for a total population of one million people suggested in the Royal College of Psychiatrists (2000) report. This staffing covers the provision for the two teams described above.

Box 22: WTE staff required for eating disorder services for a total population of one million people

Medical	
Consultant psychiatrist	1
Consultant psychotherapist	1
Specialist registrar (SpR)	1
Senior house officer (SHO)	0.5
Nurses	24
Psychologists	2
Family therapists	2
Occupational and/or creative therapists	3
Chef	0.5
Dietician	1
Secretaries	2.5
Administrator/manager	1
Total	**39.5**

4. Local personality disorder services

Services required

The document *Personality Disorder: No longer a diagnosis of exclusion* (NIMHE, 2003) recommended that service provision for personality disorder can most appropriately be provided by means of:

1. The development of a specialist multidisciplinary personality disorder team to target those with significant distress or difficulty who present with complex problems; and
2. The development of specialist day patient services in areas with high concentrations of morbidity.

Epidemiological base

Moran (2003) reviewed the epidemiology of personality disorders for the Department of Health review that led to the publication of *Personality Disorder: No longer a diagnosis of exclusion*.

Community studies of the prevalence of unspecified personality disorder (PD) report prevalence figures ranging from 10–13% (de Girolamo & Dotto, 2000). Community rates of Cluster B types (histrionic, narcissistic, antisocial and borderline personality disorders) are about 5.7%. Personality disorders are more common in younger age groups (particularly the 25–44 year age group) and equally distributed between men and women, although the sex ratio for specific types of personality disorder is variable e.g. antisocial PD is commoner among men. In psychiatric settings, the prevalence of personality disorders is probably high but difficult to quantify.

Several general points emerge from these studies:

- In general, the rate of personality disorders among psychiatric outpatients and inpatients is high, with many studies reporting a rate of greater than 50%.
- Borderline personality disorder is generally the most prevalent category in psychiatric settings.
- Personality disorders are particularly prevalent among inpatients with drug, alcohol, and eating disorders, often reported to be in excess of 70%.
- Commonly, people meeting criteria for one category of personality disorder also meet the criteria for other personality disorders. This may be a true concurrence of discrete personality disorder categories, or may represent the failure to define disorders precisely.
- There is some comorbidity between personality disorders and other mental health conditions.

In these settings people with Cluster B personality disorders attract the most attention. People with Cluster B personality disorders share the characteristic of poor impulse control and often present to hospital services when intoxicated or in crisis, threatening deliberate self-harm or aggression to others.

Given the difficulty in establishing a firm prevalence of these disorders, but knowing that many of this group will already be in contact with mental health services (or will have had past contact), the types of service considered here to be provided locally are outpatient-based assessment, a psychological therapies team and a day service team. The treatments provided should be evidence-based (Bateman & Tyrer, 2002). The teams should provide assessment and eclectic treatment and liaise with the other adult teams in the area. Sufficient seniority will exist to provide adequate skills, experience and supervision and sessional therapists trained in a range of therapies will be required. A team of at least six to seven personnel is required to make a 9 am to 5 pm day facility viable. These teams will be linked and share personnel. Box 23 shows the requirement for a population of 250,000.

Box 23: WTE staff required for a total population of 250,000 – Local personality disorder services	
Consultant psychiatrist/psychotherapist	1
Specialist registrar (SpR)	1
Clinical psychologists	2
Team leader (I grade or equivalent)	1
Deputy (G grade or equivalent)	1
Social worker	1
Nurse therapists	5
Sessional psychotherapists	3
Art (or other creative) therapist	1
Administrative support	2
Total	**18**

5. Services for deaf people

The Department of Health published *A Sign of the* Times, a consultation document concerned with the development of a national strategy for mental health services (both health and social care) for people in England who are deaf or deafblind (Department of Health, 2002g). The document covers the NSF standards for adults of working age who are deaf or deafblind. The principles of the document were:

- That national standards of mental health care apply equitably to people who are deaf.
- That the deaf community can conveniently access mental health services that are communicatively and therapeutically appropriate to their needs.
- That deaf people can play a leading role in the provision of such mental health services.

There is no evidence that deaf people have any different levels of severe psychiatric morbidity than those who are not, but may have a greater prevalence of depression and anxiety. Thus they are contained in the figures quoted earlier in this report.

The Department of Health lists specialised mental health services for the deaf in their Specialised Services National Definition set No. 22 (Department of Health, 2002h) and has recently published an implementation guide for *Sign of the Times* (NIMHE, 2005b).

For services for adults the *Sign of the Times* document took as its basis the Health Advisory Service report *Forging New Channels* (BSMHD, 1998). It recommended a strategic framework for commissioning and delivering specialised services based on a four-tier model of service provision for both children and adults:

Tier 1 – would involve the development of 'local services', including primary health care and local mental health services, aimed at improving recognition and earlier intervention.

Tier 2 – would be 'augmented local services'. This envisaged links between local mental health services and the specialist centres, with the latter providing consultation, training and information to the former. At Tier 1 and Tier 2, responsibility for individual patient management would remain with the local service.

Tier 3 – 'dispersed services provided by the very specialised services' suggested the consolidation and formalisation of current outpatient and community services provided by the three centres. At Tier 3, the specialised services would take lead responsibility for patient management, at times offering co-ordinated care with the local service.

Tier 4 – 'specialised services provided at the centres of special expertise' – concerned a continuation of the current specialised inpatient and day patient services provided by the three specialist centres.

For resources the document proposed that, as a disadvantaged group, deaf people should receive the same degree of access to health care as any other member of the population. It suggested that, where good practice exists, many of the recommendations should already be in place. Primary care trusts and mental health services were asked to consider whether their arrangements for deaf people need to be strengthened to meet the standards set out in this document and to implement these through better use of existing resources.

The document asked people to consider two options for the delivery of services at the intermediate tier:

1. Local mental health provider trusts develop services to meet the needs of their deaf community within the context of their LIT and local CAMHS development strategies.
2. The three existing specialised deaf services develop comprehensive multi-agency and multi-professional community services all over the country, and provide care co-ordination for all patients in their care.

The document suggested that those responsible for specialised mental health commissioning will need to review their investments to ensure that improvements can be delivered. It was recognised that forensic services for deaf people with mental health problems would be a significant and necessary investment and consideration is being given to the provision of central support for this purpose (they suggested beds at Rampton, which are included in our estimates).

For workforce planning and training the document recommended:

- ❖ To employ more deaf people in health and social care.
- ❖ To increase professional training opportunities for deaf people.
- ❖ To recruit and retain staff to offer specialised services.
- ❖ To map current specialist workers with the deaf people in relevant services.
- ❖ To encourage local mental health communities to include specialised services for deaf people in their local directories.
- ❖ To influence the development of a greater number of British Sign Language (BSL) interpreters to be available to health services. Regional educational confederations could be influential in the training of interpreters in co-operation with their professional organisation.

- To encourage training in deaf awareness across mental health professions in all agencies (education; health; social services; probation) in pre-registration and continuing professional development (CPD), education and training.

There are no available results of the consultation. In view of this we might assume the second option and assume that the existing staffing for the three specialised deaf services in London, Manchester and Birmingham meet the service needs and that no present increase in staff is required.

9 Standard 6
Services for carers

Standard 6
All individuals who provide regular and substantial care for a person on CPA should: ❖ have an assessment of their caring, physical and mental health needs, repeated on at least an annual basis ❖ have their own written care plan which is given to them and implemented in discussion with them. (Department of Health, 1999)

What type of service?

There is no set model for carers' services and no clear estimate of needs. It is assumed that there will be a new team covering the 250,000 catchment area which may be associated with the CMHT or local voluntary agencies (Department of Health, 2002f).

Epidemiological base

Using the estimate that there are approximately 430 people on enhanced CPA for a population of 250,000, we may assume:

75% need carer assessments (322 people)

50% of these carers will need some input at any one time (161 people)

15% need intensive input at any one time (48 people)

Those requiring intensive input will need seven hours of support worker time per week.

The estimated staffing is shown in Box 24.

Box 24: WTE staff required for a total population of 250,000 – Carers' services	
CPNs	5
Social workers	6
Support workers	8
Total	**19**

How does this compare to other estimates?

Figures from 2003 (Glover *et al.*, 2004) show that 155 LITs provided at least one dedicated carer service. Eight LITs reported providing no carer services and 11 LITs only provided these from within a mental health day or resource centre. The services available were:

280 carer support services (These were varied and included training courses, carer development workers, assessment teams, telephone helplines.)

177 carer support groups

90 services for respite and short breaks

By Spring 2006 there were 798 carer support workers in England (Centre for Mental Public Health, Durham University, 2006), which is less than half the number indicated in Box 24.

10 Standard 7
Actions necessary to reduce suicides

Standard 7

Local health and social care communities should prevent suicides by:

- ❖ promoting mental health for all, working with individuals and communities (Standard 1)
- ❖ delivering high quality primary mental health care (Standard 2)
- ❖ ensuring that anyone with a mental health problem can contact local services via the primary care team, a helpline or an A&E department (Standard 3)
- ❖ ensuring that individuals with severe and enduring mental illness have a care plan which meets their specific needs, including access to services round the clock (Standard 4)
- ❖ providing safe hospital accommodation for individuals who need it (Standard 5)
- ❖ enabling individuals caring for someone with severe mental illness to receive the support which they need to continue to care (Standard 6).

and in addition:

- ❖ support local prison staff in preventing suicides among prisoners
- ❖ ensure that staff are competent to assess the risk of suicide among individuals at greatest risk
- ❖ develop local systems for suicide audit to learn lessons and take any necessary action.

(Department of Health, 1999)

The service models to address Standard 7 were seen by the Department of Health (Department of Health, 1999) to be those set out in Standards 1–6. In addition, health and social services were to support prison staff in preventing suicide, ensure staff were competent to assess the risk of suicide and develop local systems for suicide audit.

In line with the official view, we have not therefore made any separate staffing estimates for Standard 7.

11 Staffing and cost implications

The service specifications described in this report include estimates, for a range of services, of the numbers of staff who will be needed to deliver the NSF-MH and related policies by 2010/11. This chapter pulls together these estimates in order to analyse the workforce implications at an aggregate level, i.e. across all services taken together, and makes comparisons with the numbers currently employed in adult mental health care. Building on this analysis of workforce requirements, estimates are also presented of how much total expenditure on adult mental health services will need to increase for the full implementation of current policy. The estimated requirement for additional funding is then compared with a similar projection included in the Treasury-sponsored Wanless review of long-term health spending (Wanless, 2002), and is assessed in the light of the current level of expenditure on adult mental health care and its prospective growth over the next few years.

Workforce requirements

Overall staff needs in 2010/11, shown separately for each major staff group, are shown in Box 25.

It should be noted that the figures in Box 25 do not cover all groups employed in adult mental health services. In particular, they exclude staff in management, administrative and clerical grades and those working in a range of other support services (catering staff, cleaners, property maintenance workers and so on). It has been beyond the scope of the analysis presented in this report to explore the staffing requirements for these groups in any detail and in the absence of such an assessment it is assumed that the numbers in the groups concerned bear a fixed numerical relationship to the overall numbers in the front-line groups listed above. In other words, if the total numbers of front-line staff need to increase by, say, 50% to deliver the NSF-MH by 2010/11, then by assumption the total numbers of support staff also need to increase by 50%. This is an inherently plausible assumption and its use in subsequent analysis is unlikely to introduce any significant margin of error.

The next question to be explored concerns the extent to which the estimated numbers of front-line staff needed in 2010/11 represent an increase on the numbers currently working in adult mental health services. Two main factors complicate this comparison.

First, for several of the staff groups listed, the available workforce statistics for the NHS and social services provide reliable data on the total numbers in the groups concerned but not a breakdown of these numbers by type of service. For example, it is known how many occupational therapists are employed in the NHS as a whole, but separate information is not available on how many of these are working in adult mental health services rather than in physical disability services or other areas of health provision.

Box 25: Overall staffing needs for 2010/11	
Consultant psychiatrists	4,075
Other medical staff	6,844
Qualified nurses	70,790
Social workers	10,211
Clinical psychologists	9,954
Psychological therapists (including psychotherapists and counsellors)	6,366
Occupational therapists	7,300
Pharmacists	1,286
Dieticians	676
Mental health promotion specialists	1,428
Speech/language therapists	103
Psychology assistants	2,749
Gateway workers	500
Primary care mental health workers	1,000
Pharmacy technicians	907
Employment support specialists	1,345
BME support workers	1,138
Other support workers (including 10,000 STR workers)	35,030
OT assistants	2,905
Nursing assistants	17,743
Workers for day centres	10,136

Disaggregated statistics of the type required are however available for the following: all medical staff (i.e. consultants and other medical grades), qualified nurses, social workers, clinical psychologists and psychotherapists. Taken together, these groups – arbitrarily described hereafter as the 'key clinical groups' – account for over half of all front-line staff by number and, given the preponderance of higher-paid staff in these groups, for considerably more than half the total paybill for front-line staff.

The second complication is that the estimated staff numbers for 2010/11 given here represent an overall workforce requirement for the provision of publicly funded mental health services, whether supplied by the public sector, in the form of the NHS and local authority social services departments, or by the independent and voluntary sectors providing care on a contractual basis. An appropriate comparison with the numbers of staff currently working in adult mental health services must therefore ensure that the latter include not just those directly employed by the NHS and local authorities but also those in the non-statutory sector who are providing publicly funded care. Unfortunately, comprehensive and reliable workforce statistics of the type required for the non-statutory sector are not available. It is however known from published financial data that in 2005/06 purchases of services from the non-statutory sector accounted for 17.1% of all public expenditure on adult mental health services (Mental Health Strategies, 2006) and for the purpose of subsequent analysis it is assumed here that the same ratio applies to staff numbers. In other words, for every 1000 workers, of whatever type, providing adult mental health care, 171 are assumed to be employed in the non-statutory sector and the remaining 829 in the NHS and local authorities.

Taking into account the adjustment just described, Box 26 provides a comparison between the numbers of staff working in the so-called key clinical groups in 2005/06 and the required numbers in 2010/11.

Box 26: Comparison of current and required staff numbers (all adult mental health services)

	Current numbers[1]	Required numbers
	2005/06	**2010/11**
Consultant psychiatrists	2,689	4,075
Other medical staff	4,446	6,844
Qualified nurses	51,298	70,790
Social workers	6,124	10,211
Clinical psychologists, psychotherapists and counsellors	13,623	16,320
All above groups	**78,180**	**108,240**

1 Sources: all figures for 2005/06 are taken from NHS Information Centre (2006) except for social workers (where the number is taken from Centre for Public Mental Health (2006)) and counsellors (where use is made of the estimate of 5,000 cited in Layard *et al.* (2006)), increased in each case by 20.6% (i.e. 171/829 x 100) to allow for numbers employed in the non-statutory sector.

The figures indicate that overall numbers of staff in the groups shown need to increase by 38.4% from the 2005/06 base in order to implement the NSF-MH in full by 2010/11.

Expenditure analysis

The public expenditure implications of the service specifications and associated workforce requirements described in this report could, in principle, be analysed in a number of ways. One approach would be to do a bottom-up costing, assessing how much expenditure needs to increase on a service by service basis. To give an example, Box 27 shows our estimates of the numbers of care staff who will be needed in 2010/11 in the new specialist teams proposed in the NSF-MH (assertive outreach, crisis resolution and early intervention) and compares these with the numbers currently working in the teams concerned. These figures show that, taking all specialist teams together, overall numbers of care staff need to increase by 86.4% to close the gap between the numbers currently working in these teams and the numbers needed in 2010/11.

Box 27: Comparison of required and actual numbers of care staff in specialist teams

	AOTs	CRTs	EITs	Combined
Care staff required in 2010/11	4,906	5,382	4,264	14,552
Numbers working in 2005/06	2,551	4,322	932	7,805
Required increase	**+92.3%**	**+24.5%**	**+357.5%**	**+86.4%**

The financial mapping returns for adult mental health services that are submitted each year by local implementation teams and analysed for the Department of Health by the consultancy Mental Health Strategies show that in 2005/06 total expenditure on the specialist teams amounted to £298.5 million (AOTs £101.4 million, CRTs £155.2 million and EITs £41.9 million) (Mental Health Strategies, 2006). Assuming that all other costs move in line with numbers of care staff, it can readily be estimated from the figures in Box 27 that aggregate expenditure on the specialist teams needs to rise to £556.4 million by 2010/11, an increase of £257.9 million from the level of spending in 2005/06.

A major attraction of using a bottom-up approach on the lines just described is that it would allow an assessment to be made on a service by service basis of the gap between current and required levels of spending. This would almost certainly show, for example, that some services are further away from target than others, which in turn might have important implications for the choice of spending priorities in the years ahead. Assuming that there is some merit in a reasonably balanced implementation of the various NSF-MH standards, it would be helpful to know where the distance still to be travelled is greatest and accordingly to consider the scope for focusing additional resources on these areas.

Unfortunately data shortages prevented this approach from being applied across the board. In particular, detailed information on current staff numbers was not available for a number of important individual service areas, resulting in the lack of reliable baselines against which to set our estimates of the numbers of staff required, service by service, in 2010/11. Given this absence of detailed benchmark data, a top-down approach necessarily had to be used for costing purposes.

In essence, this entailed basing our projections of expenditure on the required increase in overall staff numbers in the key clinical groups, as shown in Box 26. It has been seen that, in order to implement the NSF-MH in full by 2010/11, the total numbers in these groups need to rise by 38.4% from their current level. This estimate already includes an adjustment to allow for staff working in the non-statutory sector as well as in the NHS and local authorities, and one or two further adjustments are now required in order to convert the increase into a corresponding estimate of the requirement for total additional public spending on adult mental health services.

First, the figures in Box 26 need to be weighted to allow for differences in relative pay between the various groups. It costs more to employ an additional consultant psychiatrist than an additional nurse and, as can be seen in Box 26, the required numbers in these two groups grow at different rates. Box 28 shows the relativities that were used, based on averages of data for budgeted salaries (pay + National Insurance contributions + occupational pension contributions) for 2006 (i.e. post-Agenda for Change) kindly supplied by three leading NHS mental health trusts. The overall effect of weighting according to relative pay is to increase slightly the aggregate growth requirement between 2005/06 and 2010/11, from 38.4% to 39.7%.

Box 28: Weightings used to allow for differences in relative pay between staff groups

	Weighting
Qualified nurses	1.00
Consultant psychiatrists	3.48
Other medical staff	1.69
Clinical psychologists	1.53
Talking therapists	1.32
Social workers	1.27

Second, an adjustment is needed to allow for real increases in pay between 2005/06 and 2010/11, i.e. increases over and above general inflation. One possibility would be to ignore such increases and to show all the figures at fixed 2005/06 prices. This would however be misleading to the extent that pay increases ahead of general inflation imply a rising real economic cost of mental health care and hence a need for higher taxation to finance it. The assumption followed here is that pay in health and social services will increase relative to general inflation at its long-term historical rate. This follows the assumption made in the Wanless review of long-term health spending referred to earlier, where it is noted that the relevant increase is 2.4% a year. Pay accounts for three-quarters of total mental health service costs (Audit Commission, 2006), so if it is further assumed that prices for non-pay inputs rise at the same rate as general inflation, it can be calculated that on a weighted basis the economic cost of mental health services will increase by 1.8% a year in real terms for any given level of staff numbers. Compounded over five years, this increases the aggregate growth requirement between 2005/06 and 2010/11 from 39.7% to 52.7%.

Finally, allowance needs to be made for increases in staff numbers in groups other than those shown in Box 26 and for increases in non-pay inputs. As noted earlier, data limitations have prevented any detailed analysis of staffing changes in the groups not covered in Box 26 and it is assumed that, to deliver services effectively, the numbers of staff in these groups need to increase proportionately in line with numbers in the key clinical groups. Similarly, in the case of non-pay inputs, it is assumed that these bear a fixed or constant relationship to staff inputs and no separate calculations have been made.

The top-down costing method used here thus indicates that, for full implementation of the NSF-MH and related policies, spending on adult mental health services needs to increase between 2005/06 and 2010/11 by 52.7% in real terms. This is equivalent to an average increase of 8.8% a year in real terms. In turn, this translates into an average increase in cash or money terms of 11.5% a year, assuming general inflation of 2.5% a year.

Assessment

To the best of our knowledge, the only official published estimate of the cost of implementing the NSF-MH is given in the Wanless report *Securing Our Future Health: Taking a long-term view* (Wanless, 2002). This includes a table giving cost estimates for implementing all five disease-based NSFs that had been published up to 2002 (coronary heart disease, cancer, renal disease, mental health and diabetes). The figures are attributed to the Department of Health and show in the case of mental health that implementation of the NSF-MH would require expenditure on services for adults of working age to increase in real terms from £3.3 billion in 2002/03 to £6.4 billion in 2010/11. This is equivalent to an average real increase of 8.8% a year. The Wanless report provides no information on how this estimate was prepared nor a breakdown of projected expenditure in 2010/11 between the various NSF-MH standards or service areas.

To compare this estimate of required spending with our assessment, the former needs to be rebased so that the starting year is 2005/06 rather than 2002/03. Information from the financial mapping returns described earlier shows that between 2002/03 and 2005/06 aggregate expenditure on mental health services for adults of working age rose in cash terms by 32.2% (Mental Health Strategies, 2006). Taking into account general inflation, this represents an increase in real terms of 22.4%, or an average increase of 7.0% a year. As this is less than the required annual increase of 8.8% noted above, spending must rise at an even faster rate from 2005/06 onwards if the target level of expenditure in 2010/11 is to be achieved. Taking into account the recorded growth in spending between 2002/03 and 2005/06, expenditure up to 2010/11 now needs to increase at an average rate of 9.6% a year in real terms to deliver the NSF-MH as costed in the Wanless report. Over the five-year period as a whole, this translates into a rise in expenditure of 58.4% in real terms.

It can be seen that the required real increase in spending of 9.6% a year up to 2010/11 is broadly in line with the corresponding figure of 8.8% a year produced by our assessment. The absence of published information on the underlying basis of the Wanless calculation prevents a detailed comparison of the two estimates, but it seems clear that broadly similar conclusions have been reached concerning the overall resource requirements of the NSF-MH, particularly numbers of additional staff. This is reassuring and suggests that our estimate is reasonably robust. Indeed, our assessment of expenditure implications may if anything be on the conservative side. It remains to be considered whether additional resources for mental health are likely to be forthcoming on the scale required, having regard to past and prospective expenditure trends.

Dealing first with past increases in spending, Box 29 provides details on aggregate expenditure on mental health services for adults of working age for each year from 1999/2000 (the year in which the NSF-MH was published) to 2005/06. All figures are at 2005/06 prices, taking into account general inflation.

Box 29: Expenditure on mental health services for working-age adults[1]

Year	£ million (2005/06 prices)
1999/00	3,333
2000/01	3,573
2001/02	3,623
2002/03	4,006
2003/04	4,136
2004/05	4,615
2005/06	4,904

[1]Sources: derived from figures in Department of Health (2004a) and Mental Health Strategies (2006).

The figures show that over this period spending increased in total by 47.1% in real terms, equivalent to an average increase of 6.7% a year. This represented a substantial increase in the availability of resources for mental health and clearly allowed considerable progress to be made in improving services along the path set by the NSF-MH.

If spending continues to rise at 6.7% a year in real terms from 2005/06 onwards, it will reach £6,781 million by 2010/11. In comparison, our assessment indicates that aggregate expenditure needs to increase to £7,488 million by 2010/11 (i.e. an increase of 52.7% on the total of £4,904 million for 2005/06 shown in Box 29), while the corresponding figure implied by the Wanless estimate is £7,768 million. The continuing growth of spending on mental health services at the rate experienced since publication of the NSF-MH, rapid though this has been, would therefore still leave a shortfall in resource availability of 9.4% in relation to our assessment and 12.7% in relation to the Wanless estimate.

The spending increases for mental health shown in Box 29 occurred at a time when overall expenditure on the NHS and social services was rising particularly quickly by historical standards. Total health spending rose by 57.3% in real terms in the six years between 1999/2000 and 2005/06, a bigger increase than achieved in all of the previous 12 years combined (50.9%) (HM Treasury, 2006a). Put another way, the expenditure growth rate more than doubled. Looking ahead, it seems unrealistic to assume that spending will continue to rise at this rapid rate for all of the remaining period to 2010/11.

Departmental spending plans have already been set for 2006/07 and 2007/08 and these show that total spending on the NHS will increase by an average of 7.1% a year in real terms (HM Treasury, 2004). This is very much in line with recent trends. However, spending on local authority social services, which accounts for about a fifth of all public expenditure on adult mental health care, will rise by only 1.3% a year. Taking a weighted average of these two increases and assuming that the share of mental health in both programmes remains constant, it can be calculated that expenditure on mental health is planned to increase by 5.9% a year in real terms over the next two years.

For the three years after 2007/08, expenditure plans for individual programmes will not be announced until completion of the Comprehensive Spending Review reporting in the summer of 2007, but at the aggregate level the public finance projections published with the 2006 Budget indicate that total public spending over this period will grow at only 1.8% a year in real terms (HM Treasury, 2006b). This is well under half the average growth rate of 4.4% a year achieved between 1999/2000 and 2005/06 and even priority programmes such as the NSF-MH seem certain to be affected by the slow-down.

A possible set of assumptions is that in the three years beginning in 2008/09 total spending on the NHS will grow at half the annual rate that is planned for 2006/07 and 2007/08, i.e. 3.55% a year in real terms, and total spending on social services will grow at the same rate as planned for these two years, i.e. 1.3% a year. On the further assumption that mental health maintains a constant share in both these programmes, the end-result is a projection that expenditure on mental health services will increase by 3.1% a year in real terms in the last three years of the NSF-MH planning period. As with public spending generally, this is less than half the annual growth rate achieved over the period 1999/2000 to 2005/06. It may also be optimistic, for example in assuming that mental health maintains a constant spending share. The historical record shows that while total health expenditure increased by 57.3% in real terms between 1999/2000 and 2005/06, spending on adult mental health services rose by 47.1%, in other words a declining share.

Bringing together the planned increases for 2006/07 and 2007/08 and the projected increases for the following three years, the scenario suggested here is that over the five-year period to 2010/11 spending on mental health will increase by 22.0% in real terms, to £6,027 million by the end of the period. This is a shortfall of 19.5% relative to the expenditure requirement given by our assessment and 22.4% relative to the Wanless estimate. Put another way, in 2010/11 funded capacity for adult mental health care is likely to be at around 80% of its target level.

12 Conclusions

This report has sought to specify and cost a service for working-age adults in England that delivers the Government's key policy objectives for mental health, in particular the *National Service Framework for Mental Health* (Department of Health, 1999).

The report is forward-looking, in line with the planned ten-year timescale for implementation of the NSF-MH. It describes a set of services, and their associated resource requirements, that are required by 2010/11. The findings raise a series of important questions: what remains to be done over the next few years to secure achievement of the NSF-MH standards? What does this imply for the balance and configuration of services and the size of the workforce, and how much will it cost?

In addition the analysis has a variety of potential uses, locally and nationally, in the planning and design of individual services and in more aggregate applications such as budgeting, workforce planning, policy monitoring and system reform.

Services – configuration and balance

The specification of the service models required to deliver policy objectives varies from service to service in the policy documents that we have examined. For standards 4 and 5, official guidance is detailed and prescriptive in its description of the new specialist community teams but not in relation to hospital inpatient services. It does not reach this level of specification for any of the other standards. The services required for standard 1, on health promotion, are not well defined in official policy statements and little else exists to help us to specify the types or models of services that should make up our approach to mental health promotion. Whilst it is acknowledged that much of this may be attained by cross-cutting government policies, there is still a need to house specific initiatives in health and social services.

For primary care (standards 2 and 3), we have not prescribed any model of service but have rather focused on specific medication needs and the number of therapists required to provide psychological therapies for people with depression and anxiety. This is in line with the aspirations set out in the Government's five-year review of the NSF-MH to improve access to psychological therapies and the recent CBT pilots. However, the actual delivery and organisation of these services for primary care have not been specified, although some models have been suggested elsewhere (The Sainsbury Centre for Mental Health, 2006). More detailed policy initiatives are required in this area as well as piloting of any proposed models of delivery and testing of the application of psychological therapies in actual practice.

Within the secondary services (standards 4 and 5), three aspects of care delivery warrant further attention. The first is rehabilitation, where there are no current policy initiatives for the development of services. The focus on acute care and risk containment may be partly responsible for this neglect.

The second is the provision of services that help to promote the social inclusion of people with mental health problems. Some of these may be related to standard 1, but others are concerned with standards 4 and 5 and the appropriate day and vocational services. The final area relates to the overlap of traditionally non-adult services and patient groups and those traditionally seen to be the province of working-age adult mental health services. The groups concerned include adolescents and young adults, people with learning difficulties and those with autism spectrum disorders and people with alcohol and drug misuse problems. These groups are often poorly served by the existing services and fall between the gaps at the interfaces.

Research and development

One rationale used in this report and in the NSF-MH for including and specifying services is the existence of evidence to support their use. For many of the new community teams there is some backing from systematic reviews (Marshall & Lockwood, 1998; Marshall *et al.*, 1998; Catty *et al.*, 2002; Joy *et al.*, 1998; Simmons *et al.*, 2001); the use of psychological therapies and medication is also supported by systematically appraised evidence (e.g. NICE, 2002; 2004a; 2004b; 2006). However there has been no systematic research programme examining the implementation of the NSF-MH. In particular, what is the effect of introducing the new community teams (assertive outreach, crisis resolution and early intervention)? How do these fit with the generic community mental health teams (CMHTs): does this approach provide effective and efficacious delivery of community-based mental health care? Also, how does this provision balance with other services including inpatient units, day care and primary care? We may have missed an opportunity to monitor and assess the implementation of these teams and their effect on the delivery of local services for people with severe mental illness and those with more prevalent forms of disorders.

Staffing

The effective delivery of mental health care is highly dependent on the availability of sufficient numbers of appropriately trained staff. Mental health services use a central core of professionally affiliated staff who increasingly have been organised into multi-professional teams. The use of such staff promotes expertise, training, professional standards and accountability, all of which are expected by the public. In addition, non-professionally affiliated staff, particularly support workers, are required to supplement the work of the professional groups. These staff are often highly regarded by users, but still require training, supervision and quality assurance. The actual balance of professional and non-professionally affiliated staff, as well as the proportions of the different types of professional staff, may be debated, but we believe that by using current patterns of staff groups and by emphasising the needs of the services and their users, we have provided a clear rationale for our assessments of workforce needs. What is clear is that there is a need to increase the numbers of staff in all groups. Across all services, we estimate that delivery of the NSF-MH and related policies requires aggregate staff numbers to increase by nearly 40% between 2005/06 and 2010/11. We have not addressed the way in which staff execute their roles or their ways of working together. These matters have been discussed separately in *New Ways of Working* (Department of Health, 2005b)

Resource requirements

It is clear from our analysis that the NSF-MH set a very ambitious agenda for the provision of better services. Views may differ on exactly what needs to be done to deliver the NSF-MH standards in full, but there is little doubt that the resource requirements are substantial. Taking 1999/2000 (the year in which the NSF-MH was published) as a baseline, our assessment suggests that over the whole period to 2010/11 spending would need to increase by about 125% in real terms (the official estimate quoted in the Wanless report implies an even larger increase, of around 133%). This is equivalent to an average rise in expenditure of 7.6% a year in real terms, to be sustained – year in, year out – over a full decade.

Figures presented in the previous chapter show that between 1999/2000 and 2005/06 the actual growth in spending on mental health services averaged 6.7% a year in real terms, not far short of the required rate. This was a major achievement and undoubtedly allowed substantial progress, in terms of more and better services, along the path set by the NSF-MH.

Looking ahead, it seems unrealistic to assume that the expenditure growth rates of the recent past can be sustained over the remainder of the period to 2010/11. In the short term the NHS is grappling with a number of financial pressures from which mental health services are not immune. In the later years of the period, current plans are for a substantial slow-down in the growth of public spending as a whole and again mental health cannot expect to be exempt. According to a plausible projection for spending on mental health services suggested in the previous chapter, the overall availability of resources in 2010/11 is likely to be, in very broad terms, about 20% short of the level required for full implementation of the NSF-MH and related policies.

Final questions and future vision

This prospective funding gap should not necessarily be interpreted as a criticism or as a sign of failure but rather as a measure of the very ambitious nature of the agenda for the development of mental health services that was launched by the NSF-MH. In 1999, the NSF-MH provided a clear statement of the future direction of mental health services, contributed to the status of an area previously regarded as a Cinderella discipline, put the services in line with other health priorities and linked them with new funding. It was received with a broad consensus of agreement, which acknowledged the post-war developments of the move away from asylum care and the expansion of community-based services. When the NSF-MH was published at the end of the twentieth century the building blocks for community services were in place, but were under-developed and under-resourced and in need of strategic direction, modernisation and a firm funding base. The resource implications of the NSF-MH were not explicitly stated at the time, but it is clear from our estimates and those given in the Wanless report (2002) that they were very substantial.

The likely shortfall in funding for 2010/11 noted above raises some important, multi-layered questions for debate about priorities for the future and the distribution of resources across England. If, as seems likely, resources for mental health become increasingly constrained over the next few years and not all the objectives of the NSF-MH can be delivered within the planned timescale, how should any extra money be most sensibly used? This question needs to be set against an ever-changing pattern of development. Services themselves are evolving, as is the evidence that supports them. For example, questions have been asked about the appropriate role of assertive outreach teams and the future use of these teams may require a change in emphasis or a shift in policy. The adoption of new technologies such as the atypical antipsychotics or computerised methods of psychological therapy will require increased spending in these areas. The need for improvement in the fabric of inpatient units will increase capital costs. New service needs, such as for asylum seekers, an increasingly culturally diverse population and an increase in substance misuse, will place additional burdens on services. The increasing demand for talking therapies increases the need for trained therapists to deliver these. There is, as yet, no agreement as to the number of forensic beds required and the cost of forensic services is likely to grow. Other components of policy may provide difficult challenges for mental health services, such as increasing patient choice or implementing change to the Mental Health Act.

This report has not offered a vision for future services, preferring to leave this to others (The Sainsbury Centre for Mental Health, 2006; Rankin, 2005). However, there is a vision of services implicit in those aspects of policy that promote social inclusion, citizenship and rights. These principles are not merely abstract, but are central to the lives of current and potential service users. Issues still to be resolved concern the availability of sufficient resources to match the vision and the nature of the longer-term strategy to secure an equitable distribution of these resources. This report has analysed the resource inputs necessary to deliver the policy aspirations, but what progress has been made in delivering improved outcomes for mental health services and users? Some NSF-MH standards have advanced more than others, but what of those standards that lag behind? Against this background, what review of policy should be conducted between now and 2010/11? What priorities should government policy be setting as the life-span of the NSF-MH draws to a close? Will there be an NSF-MH Mark 2 and what form should this take?

With these questions in mind we believe that a clear policy direction for mental health services needs to be developed and maintained. Modern mental health services are relatively new and have been tested out over the past six to seven years through progress on some of the NSF-MH standards. An overview of this progress is urgently needed and work should be commissioned to evaluate the effects of the new community teams and their consequences for the broader system, as well as assessing the gaps in attainment of the NSF-MH standards. Priorities must be set for the remaining years of the NSF-MH up to 2010/11. There needs to be a clear commitment by the Government to do the preparatory work, starting now, that is necessary to create the plans for mental health services after 2010/11. In the light of our review this requires the formulation of a clear view of the future direction, standards, delivery and structure of twenty-first century mental health services, along with a published analysis of the implications for staffing and other resources.

Taking a longer and broader perspective, we acknowledge that a great deal has been achieved over the post-war period in developing a modern mental health service in this country, one that is at the forefront of international good practice. Nevertheless, much remains to be done, particularly in building an inclusive system that puts people with mental health problems at its heart. The NHS spending environment is currently constrained and is likely to remain so, which may result in the declared priority status of mental health being put under increasing strain. Having made so much progress up to now, this would be a backward step. We strongly believe that a successor to the NSF-MH is needed to maintain the momentum of recent years.

References

Abraham, C. & Michie, S. (2005) Contributing to public health policy and practice. *The Psychologist*, **18**, 676–679.

Audit Commission (2002) *A Spoonful of Sugar: Medicines' management in NHS hospitals.* Wetherby: Audit Commission Publications.

Audit Commission (2006) *Managing Finances in Mental Health.* London: Audit Commission.

Bateman & Tyrer (2002) *Effective Management of Personality Disorder.* (Paper commissioned to support the publication NIMHE (2003) *Personality disorder. No longer a diagnosis of exclusion. Policy implementation guidance for the development of services for people with personality disorder.* London: Department of Health (http://kc.nimhe.org.uk/upload/Bateman%20&%20Tyrer.doc) [Accessed 12 December 2006]

Boardman, J. (2005) New Services for Old – An overview of mental health policy. In: Bell, A. & Lindley, P. (eds) *Beyond the Water Towers. The unfinished revolution in mental health services 1985–2005.* London: The Sainsbury Centre for Mental Health.

Boardman, J. & Parsonage, M. (2005) *Defining a Good Mental Health Service. A discussion paper.* London: The Sainsbury Centre for Mental Health (Web paper).

Boardman, J., Willmott, S. & Henshaw, C. (2004) The prevalence of the needs for mental health treatment in general practice attenders. *British Journal of Psychiatry*, **185**, 318–327.

Borrill, J., Maden, A., Martin, A., Weaver, T., Stimson., G., Farrell, M. & Barnes, T. (2003) *Differential substance misuse treatment needs of women, ethnic minorities and young offenders in prison: prevalence of substance misuse and treatment needs.* Home Office Online Report Series. (http://www.homeoffice.gov.uk/rds/pdfs2/rdsolr3303.pdf) [Accessed 12 December 2006]

British Psychological Society (2004) *Estimating the applied psychology demand in adult mental health.* Leicester: British Psychological Society.

BSMHD British Society for Mental Health and Deafness (1998) *Forging new channels. Commissioning and delivering mental health services for people who are deaf. An NHS health advisory service thematic review.* London: Health Advisory Service.

Buchan, J. & Dal Poz, M. R. (2002) Skill Mix in the Health Care Workforce: Reviewing the Evidence. *Bulletin of the World Health Organisation*, **80**, 7.

Buchan, J., Ball, J. & O'May, F. (2000) Determining Skill Mix in the Health Workforce: Guidelines for Managers and Health Professionals. *Issues in Health Services Delivery, Paper Number 3.* Department of Organisation of Health Services Delivery. Geneva: World Health Organisation.

Bullock, T. (2003) Changing levels of drug use before, during and after imprisonment. In: Ramsey, M. (ed) *Prisoners' Drug Use and Treatment: Seven Research Studies.* Home Office Research Study 267. London: Home Office Research, Development and Statistics Directorate.

Catty, J., Burns, T. & Knapp, M. *et al.* (2002) Home treatment for mental health problems: a systematic review. *Psychological Medicine,* **32**, 383–401.

Centre for Public Mental Health, Durham University (2006) *Adult Mental Health Service Mapping: Reporting Autumn 2004 and Spring 2006.* (www.amhmapping.org.uk/reports/) [Accessed 5 December 2006]

Citizens Advice Bureau (2005) *Prescribing Advice: Improving health through CAB advice services.* CAB Summer 2005. London: CAB.

Confidential Enquiry into Maternal and Child Health (2004) *Why Mothers Die 2000–2002. The Sixth Report of Confidential Enquiries into Maternal Deaths in the United Kingdom.* London: Royal College of Obstetricians and Gynaecologists.

Cox, C. R. (2004) *Determining Nursing Establishment and Grade Mix in Psychiatric Inpatient Wards.* Report from Avon and Wiltshire Partnership NHS Trust. Unpublished.

Crowther, R.E. & Marshall, M. (2001) Employment rehabilitation schemes for people with mental health problems in the North West Region: Service characteristics and utilisation. *Journal of Mental Health,* **10**, 373–382.

Crowther, R.E, Marshall, M., Bond, G.R. & Huxley, P. (2001) Helping people with severe mental illness to obtain work: systematic review. *British Medical Journal,* **322**, 204–208.

Department of Health (1997) *The New NHS: Modern, Dependable.* CM3807. London: HMSO.

Department of Health (1998a) *Modernising Mental Health Services: Safe Sound and Supportive.* London: Department of Health.

Department of Health (1998b) *Our Healthier Nation: A Contract for Health.* CM3852. London: HMSO.

Department of Health (1998c) *Modernising Social Services: Promoting independence, improving projection, raising standards.* CM4169. London: Department of Health.

Department of Health (1998d) *A First Class Service: Quality in the New NHS.* London: Department of Health.

Department of Health (1998e) *Working Together: Securing a Quality Workforce for the NHS.* London: Department of Health.

Department of Health (1999) *National Service Framework for Mental Health: Modern Standards and Service Models.* London: Department of Health.

Department of Health (2000a) *The NHS Plan: A Plan for Investment. A Plan for Reform.* CM4818–I. London: Department of Health.

Department of Health (2000b) *Pharmacy in the Future: Implementing the NHS Plan.* London: Department of Health.

Department of Health (2000c) *Shaping the Future NHS: Long-term planning for hospitals and related services consultation document on the findings of The National Beds Inquiry – supporting analysis.* London: Department of Health.

Department of Health (2001a) *Mental Health Policy Implementation Guide*. London: Department of Health.

Department of Health (2001b) *Mental Health National Service Framework (and NHS Plan) Workforce planning, education and training, underpinning programme: adult mental health services. Final report by the Workforce Action Team*. London: Department of Health.

Department of Health (2001c) *The Expert Patient: A New Approach to Chronic Disease Management for the 21st Century*. London: Department of Health.

Department of Health (2001d) *The National Institute for Mental Health in England: Role and Function*. London: Department of Health.

Department of Health (2001e) *The National Service Framework for Diabetes: Standards*. London: Department of Health.

Department of Health (2002a) *Community Mental Health Teams: Policy Implementation Guide*. London: Department of Health.

Department of Health (2002b) *Mental Health Policy Implementation Guide: Adult Acute Inpatient Care Provision*. London: Department of Health.

Department of Health (2002c) *Mental Health Policy Implementation Guide: Dual Diagnosis Good Practice Guide*. London: Department of Health.

Department of Health (2002d) *Mental Health Policy Implementation Guide: National Minimum Standards for General Adult Services in Psychiatric Intensive Care Units (PICU) and Low Secure Environments*. London: Department of Health.

Department of Health (2002e) *Women's Mental Health: Into the Mainstream: Draft Strategy*. London: Department of Health.

Department of Health (2002f) *Developing Services for Carers and Families of People with Mental Illness*. London: Department of Health.

Department of Health (2002g) *A Sign of the Times: Modernising Mental Health Services for People who are Deaf (consultation)*. London: Department of Health.

Department of Health (2002h) *Specialised Services National Definition Set: 22. Specialised Mental Health (adult)*. London: Department of Health.

Department of Health (2003a) *Mental Health Policy Implementation Guide: Support, Time and Recovery (STR) Workers*. London: Department of Health.

Department of Health (2003b) *Mainstreaming Gender and Women's Mental Health: Implementation guidance*. London: Department of Health.

Department of Health (2003c) *Fast Forwarding Primary Care Mental Health, Graduate Primary Care Mental Health Workers: Best practice guidance*. London: Department of Health.

Department of Health (2003d) *Fast Forwarding Primary Care Mental Health, 'Gateway' Workers: Guidance*. London: Department of Health.

Department of Health (2003e) *Delivering Race Equality: A Framework for Action in Mental Health Services. Consultation Document*. London: Department of Health.

Department of Health (2003f) *Payment by Results: Preparing for 2005*. London: Department of Health.

Department of Health (2003g) *Short Guide to NHS Foundation Trusts*. London: Department of Health.

Department of Health (2004a) *The National Service Framework for Mental Health – Five years on*. London: Department of Health.

Department of Health (2004b) *Policy Implementation Guide. Community Development Workers for Black and Minority Ethnic Communities. Interim Guidance*. London: Department of Health.

Department of Health (2004c) *Developing Positive Practice to Support the Safe and Therapeutic Management of Aggression and Violence in Mental Health Inpatient Settings: Mental Health Policy Implementation Guide*. London: Department of Health.

Department of Health (2004d) *Improving Mental Health Law. Towards a new Mental Health Act*. London: Department of Health

Department of Health (2004e) *Mental Health Care Group Workforce Team: National Mental Health Workforce Strategy*. London: Department of Health.

Department of Health (2004f) *The NHS Improvement Plan: Putting People at the Heart of Public Services*. London: The Stationery Office.

Department of Health (2004g) *Practice Based Commissioning: Promoting Clinical Engagement*. London: Department of Health.

Department of Health (2004h) *Choosing Health: Making Healthier Choices Easier. Public Health White Paper*. London: Department of Health.

Department of Health (2004i) *Standards for Better Health*. London: Department of Health.

Department of Health (2004j) *Building a Safer NHS for Patients: Improving Medication Safety*. London: Department of Health.

Department of Health (2004k) *The Ten Essential Shared Capabilities: A Framework for the Whole of the Mental Health Workforce*. London: Department of Health.

Department of Health (2004l) *Children, Young People and Maternity Services National Service Framework*. London: Department of Health.

Department of Health (2005a) *Delivering race equality in mental health care: An action plan for reform inside and outside services and the Government's response to the Independent Inquiry into the death of David Bennett*. London: Department of Health.

Department of Health (2005b) *New Ways of Working for Psychiatrists: Enhancing effective, person-centred services through new ways of working in multi-disciplinary and multi-agency contexts. Final Report July 2005 "but not the end of the story"*. London: Department of Health.

Department of Health (2005c) *Creating a Patient-led NHS: Delivering the NHS Improvement Plan*. London: Department of Health.

Department of Health (2005d) *Supporting People with Long-term Conditions: an NHS and Social Care Model to support local innovation and integration*. London: Department of Health.

Department of Health (2005e) *National Service Framework for Long-term Conditions*. London: Department of Health.

Department of Health (2005f) *Improving Mental Health Services by Extending the Role of Nurses in Prescribing and Supplying Medication*. London: Department of Health.

Department of Health (2005g) *Independence, Well-being and Choice: Our Vision for the Future of Social Care for Adults in England*. CM6499. (Social Care Green Paper). London: The Stationery Office.

Department of Health (2006a) *From Segregation to Inclusion: Commissioning Guidance on Day Services for People with Mental Health Problems*. London: Department of Health.

Department of Health (2006b) *Supporting Women into the Mainstream. Commissioning Women-only Community Day Services*. London: Department of Health.

Department of Health (2006c) *The Mental Health Bill. Plans to amend the Mental Health Act 1983. Briefing sheet. Implementing Government Policies on Mental Health Law*. London: Department of Health.

Department of Health (2006d) *Health Reform in England: Update and Commissioning Framework*. London: Department of Health.

Department of Health (2006e) *Choosing Health: Supporting the Physical Health Needs of People with Severe Mental Illness: Commissioning Framework*. London: Department of Health.

Department of Health/Department for Work and Pensions (2006) *Vocational Services for People with Severe Mental Health Problems: Commissioning Guidance*. London: Department of Health.

Department of Health/HM Prison Service (2001) *Changing the Outlook: A Strategy for Developing and Modernising Mental Health Services in Prisons*. London: Department of Health

Department for Work and Pensions (2004) *Building Capacity for Work: A UK Framework for Vocational Rehabilitation*. London: Department for Work and Pensions.

de Girolamo, G. & Dotto, P. (2000) Epidemiology of Personality Disorders. In: Gelder, M.G., Lopez-Ibor, J.J. & Andreasen, N.C. (eds) *New Oxford Textbook of Psychiatry, vol. 1*. New York: Oxford University Press.

Fender, A. (2004) *High Secure Hospital Bed Projections*. Report for Department of Health.

Gilbody, S., Whitty, P., Grimshaw, J. *et al.* (2003) Educational and organisational interventions to improve the management of depression in primary care: a systematic review. *Journal of the American Medical Association*, **289**, 3145–3151.

Glover, G., Barnes, D., Wistow, R. & Bradley, S. (2004) *Mental Health Service Provision for Working-age Adults in England 2003*. Durham: University of Durham Centre for Public Mental Health. (www.dur.ac.uk/service.mapping/amh/)

Government Actuary's Department (2006) *Population Projections*. (www.gad.gov.uk/Population_projections_background.htm) [Accessed 5 December 2006]

Grove, B. & Drurie, S. (1999) *Social Firms – An instrument for economic empowerment and inclusion*. Redhill: Social Firms UK.

HM Government (2005a) *Health, work and well-being – Caring for our future. A strategy for the health and well-being of working-age people*. London: The Stationery Office.

HM Government (2005b) *Department for Work and Pensions Five Year Strategy: Opportunity and Security throughout Life*. CM6447. London: The Stationery Office.

HM Government (2006) *A New Deal for Welfare: Empowering people to work.* (Green Paper) CM6730. London: The Stationery Office.

HM Prison Service (2001) *Prevention of Suicide and Self-harm in the Prison Service: An internal review.* (www.hmprisonservice.gov.uk/resourcecentre/publicationsdocuments) [Accessed 2 November 2005]

HM Prison Service (2005) *Population Bulletin Monthly, September 2005.* (www.hmprisonservice.gov.uk/assets/documents/10001317pop_bull_sep_05.doc) [Accessed 12 December 2006]

HM Treasury (2004) *Stability and security and opportunity for all: investing for Britain's long-term future: New public spending plans 2005–2008.* London: HM Treasury.

HM Treasury (2006a) *Public expenditure statistical analyses 2006.* London: HM Treasury. (www.hm-treasury.gov.uk)

HM Treasury (2006b) *Financial statement and budget report.* London: HM Treasury.

Home Office (2005) *Updated and revised prison population projections 2005–2011. England and Wales 10/05.* Home Office Statistical Bulletin. London: Home Office. (www.homeoffice.gov.uk/rds/pdfs05/hosb1005.pdf) [Accessed 12 December 2006]

House, A. & G., Hodgson (1994) Estimating needs and meeting demands. In: S., Benjamin, A., House & P., Jenkins (eds) *Liaison Psychiatry: defining needs and planning services.* London: Gaskell Press.

Joy, C.B., Adams, C.E. & Rice, K. (1998) *Crisis intervention for those with severe mental illness.* Database of Systematic Reviews, 2006 (www.cochrane.org/reviews) [Accessed 12 December 2006]

Laing & Buisson (2006) *Mental Health and Specialist Care Services. UK Marketing Report 2006.* London: Laing & Buisson

Layard, R. (2005) *Mental Health: Britain's biggest social problem?* Paper delivered to Cabinet Office. (www.strategy.gov.uk/seminars/mental_health/index.asp)

Layard, R. (2006) The Case for Psychological Treatment Centres. *British Medical Journal,* **332**, 1030–1032.

Layard, R., Clark, D., Knapp, M. & Mayraz, G. (2006) *Implementing the NICE guidelines for depression and anxiety: a cost-benefit analysis.* London: Centre for Economic Performance, London School of Economics. (http://cep.lse.ac.uk/research/mentalhealth/default.asp)

Litiano, S. & Ramsey, M. (2003) Prisoners' drug use before prison and the links with crime. In: Ramsey, M. (ed) *Prisoners' Drug Use and Treatment: Seven Research Studies.* Home Office Research Study 267. London: Home Office Research, Development and Statistics Directorate.

Marshall, M. & Lockwood, A. (1998) *Assertive Community Treatment for People with Severe Mental Illness.* Database of Systematic Reviews, 2006. (www.cochrane.org/reviews) [Accessed 12 December 2006]

Marshall, M., Lockwood, A. & Green, R. *et al.* (1998) *Case Management for People with Severe Mental Disorder.* Database of Systematic Reviews, 2006 (www.cochrane.org/reviews) [Accessed 12 December 2006]

Mind (2004) *Report to National Institute of Mental Health in England. Rural proofing of the National Framework for Mental Health.* London: Mind.

Meltzer, H., Gill, B., Petticrew, M. & Hinds, K. (1995) *The prevalence of psychiatric morbidity among adults living in private households. OPCS Surveys of Psychiatric Morbidity in Great Britain. Report No. 1.* OPCS, Social Survey Division. London: HMSO.

mentality (2005) *England – The country story for mental health promotion.* London: **mentality**.

Mental Aftercare Association (2002) *Changing Light Bulbs? Research into the Role of Mental Health Support Workers in East Suffolk.* London: Mental Aftercare Association.

Mental Health Strategies (2006) *The 2005/06 national survey of investment in mental health services.* London: Department of Heath.

Moran, P. (2003) *The Epidemiology of Personality Disorders* NIMHE [Paper commissioned to support the publication of NIMHE (2003) *Personality disorder. No longer a diagnosis of exclusion: policy implementation guidance for the development of services for people with personality disorder*]. London: Department of Health.

Murphy, G.H., Harnett, H. & Holland, A.J. (1995) A survey of intellectual disabilities amongst men on remand in prison. *Mental Handicap Research,* **8**, 81–98.

Murray, A., Shepherd, G., Onyett, S. & Muijen, M. (1997) *More than a Friend: Role of Support Workers in Community Mental Health Services.* London: The Sainsbury Centre for Mental Health.

NHS Information Centre (2006) *NHS Hospital and Community Staff (HCHS): Medical and Dental England 1995–2005.* (www.ic.nhs.uk/pubs/nhsstaff) [Accessed 5 December 2006]

NICE (2002) *Schizophrenia: Core interventions in the treatment and management of schizophrenia in primary and secondary care.* London: NICE.

NICE (2004a) *Anxiety: Management of anxiety disorder (panic disorder, with or without agoraphobia and generalized anxiety disorder) in adults in primary, secondary and community care.* London: NICE.

NICE (2004b) *Depression: Management of depression in primary and secondary care.* London: NICE.

NICE (2006) *Bipolar Disorder: The management of bipolar disorder in adults, children and adolescents, in primary and secondary care.* London: NICE.

NIMHE (2003) *Personality Disorder: No longer a diagnosis of exclusion. Policy implementation guidance for the development of services for people with personality disorder.* London: Department of Health.

NIMHE (2005a) *Caseload Profiling Tool v7* (www.nimhesw.nhs.uk/-Caseload Profiling Tool (v7)) [Accessed 7 June 2006]

NIMHE (2005b) *Mental Health and Deafness: Towards Equity and Access. Best Practice Guidance.* Leeds: NIMHE.

Office of Deputy Prime Minister (2004) *What is Supporting People?* London: Office of Deputy Prime Minister.

Rankin, J. (2005) *Mental Health in the Mainstream.* London: IPPR.

Rethink (2004) *Lost and Found. Voices from the forgotten generation.* London: Rethink.

Rethink (2005) *Action Stations. The way out for the forgotten generation.* London: Rethink.

Roth, A. & Fonagy, P. (2004) *What Works for Whom? A critical review of psychotherapy research.* 2nd Edition. London: Guildford Press.

Royal College of Psychiatrists (2000) *Eating Disorders in the UK.* Council Report CR87. London: Royal College of Psychiatrists.

Royal College of Psychiatrists (2005) *Prison Psychiatry; Adult Prisons in England and Wales.* London: Royal College of Psychiatrists

Royal College of Psychiatrists (2006) *Perinatal Maternal Mental Health Services.* Council Report CR88. London: Royal College of Psychiatrists.

Royal College of Psychiatrists/Royal College of Physicians (2003) *The Psychosocial Care of Medical Patients. A Practical Guide.* London: Royal College of Psychiatrists.

The Sainsbury Centre for Mental Health (1998) *Keys to Engagement: Review of Care for People with Severe Mental Illness who are hard to engage with Services.* London: The Sainsbury Centre for Mental Health.

The Sainsbury Centre for Mental Health (2003) *Money for Mental Health: A Review of Public Spending on Mental Health Care.* London: The Sainsbury Centre for Mental Health.

The Sainsbury Centre for Mental Health (2005) *The Neglected Majority: Developing Intermediate Mental Health Care in Primary Care.* London: The Sainsbury Centre for Mental Health.

The Sainsbury Centre for Mental Health (2006) *The Future of Mental Health: A Vision for 2015.* London: The Sainsbury Centre for Mental Health.

Scott, J. (2006) Depression should be managed like a chronic disease. *British Medical Journal,* **332**, 985–986.

Secretary of State for Health (2003) *Building on the Best: Choice, Responsiveness and Equity in the NHS.* CM6079. London: The Stationery Office.

Secretary of State for Health (2006) *Our Health, Our Care, Our Say: A new direction for community services.* (White Paper) CM6737. London: The Stationery Office.

Simmonds, S., Coid, J., Joseph, P., Marriott, S. & Tyrer, P. (2001) Community mental health management in severe mental illness: a systematic review. *British Journal of Psychiatry,* **178**, 497–502.

Simon, G. & von Korff, M. (1995) Recognition, management and outcomes of depression in primary care. *Archives of Family Medicine,* **4**, 99–105.

Singleton, N., Bumpstead, R., O'Brien, M., Lee, A. & Meltzer, H. (2001) *Psychiatric Morbidity among Adults living in Private Households, 2000: Summary Report.* London: Office for National Statistics.

Singleton, N. & Lewis, G. (eds) (2003) *Better or Worse: A longitudinal study of the mental health of adults living in private households in Great Britain.* London: The Stationery Office.

Singleton, N., Meltzer, H. & Gatward, R. (1998) *Psychiatric morbidity among prisoners in England and Wales.* London: The Stationery Office.

Social Exclusion Unit (2004) *Mental Health and Social Exclusion.* London: Office of the Deputy Prime Minister.

von Korff, M. & Goldberg, D. (2001) Improving Outcomes in Depression. *British Medical Journal*, **325**, 925.

Wanless, D. (2002) *Securing our Future Health: Taking a long-term view. Final Report*. London: HM Treasury.

Warr, J. (1995) Skill Mix Fixed. *Nursing Management*, **1**, (8), 11.

Wardle, J. & Steptoe, A. (2005) Public Health Psychology. *The Psychologist*, **18**, 672–675.